diabetes
DeMYSTiFieD

Demystified Series

diabetes
DeMYSTiFieD

Umesh Masharani, M.D.

New York Chicago San Francisco Lisbon London Madrid Mexico City
Milan New Delhi San Juan Seoul Singapore Sydney Toronto

Library of Congress Cataloging-in-Publication Data

Masharani, Umesh.
    Diabetes demystified : a self-teaching guide / Umesh Masharani.
        p.   cm. — (Demystified)
    ISBN-13: 978-0-07-147795-6 (alk. paper)
    ISBN-10: 0-07-147795-0 (alk. paper)
    1. Diabetes—Popular works.   I. Title.

  RC660.4.M364   2007
  616.4′62—dc22   2007030610

1 2 3 4 5 6 7 8 9 10 11 12 13 14 15 16 17 18 19 FGR/FGR 0 9 8 7

ISBN 978-0-07-147795-6
MHID   0-07-147795-0

McGraw-Hill books are available at special quantity discounts to use as premiums and sales promotions, or for use in corporate training programs. For more information, please write to the Director of Special Sales, Professional Publishing, McGraw-Hill, Two Penn Plaza, New York, NY 10121-2298. Or contact your local bookstore.

The information contained in this book is intended to provide helpful and informative material on the subject addressed. It is not intended to serve as a replacement for professional medical advice or treatment. Any use of the information in this book is at the reader's discretion. The author and publisher disclaim any and all liability arising directly or indirectly from the use or application of any information contained in this book.

This book is printed on acid-free paper.

To Nisha, Vijay, and Hansha

CONTENTS

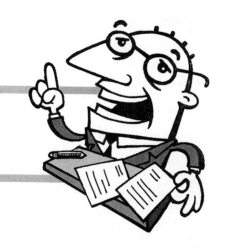

PART THREE ADDITIONAL CONSIDERATIONS

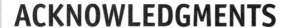

ACKNOWLEDGMENTS

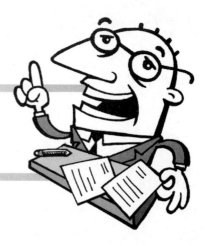

I would like to thank my colleagues at the University of California, San Francisco, who have helped shape my approach to the practice of diabetes. I am indebted to my patients, who over the years have taught me much about diabetes. Two of my diabetes educator colleagues, Marlene Bedrich and Gloria Yee, also deserve my thanks for reviewing some of the chapters and providing helpful comments about the manuscript. I would like to give a special thank-you to my editor at McGraw Hill, Johanna Bowman, for guiding and encouraging me throughout the writing of this book, and to Terre Stouffer for her careful and meticulous editorial help. Lastly, I would like to thank my wife, Hansha, for her love and support.

INTRODUCTION

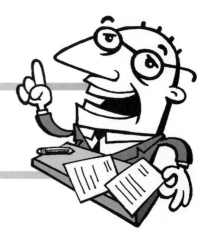

Chances are that you have picked up this book because you or someone you love has just been diagnosed with diabetes or has had diabetes for a while and you are trying to understand the disease and how to take care of it. Like all medical conditions you may find the language, medicines, and treatment recommendations complicated and confusing. You may also have heard that diabetes can cause blindness, nerve damage, or kidney failure, and you may be fearful that this could happen to you. It is true that these complications can occur if the diabetes is untreated or poorly controlled. With good care, however, all of these complications can be prevented.

The goal of this book is to demystify diabetes and give you a clear picture of what it is and how it is treated. Living with diabetes can be challenging. It demands your attention several times a day, and you cannot ignore it for long. You have to acquire a new set of skills—learning to adjust medicines, diet, and physical activity. For individuals who are very organized, the adjustments demanded by diabetes are easily incorporated into their routines. For others, the diabetes can become a straightjacket, but it does not have to be this way—there is a lot that you can do to make your diabetes manageable. This book describes how you can acquire the skills necessary to incorporate diabetes care into your daily life without feeling overwhelmed.

It may seem hard to believe, but there can be some positive aspects to a diagnosis of diabetes. First, unlike many other chronic illnesses, you can be in charge and you can control it. Second, the organizational skills and discipline that you develop caring for your diabetes can be successfully transferred to other aspects of your life. Third, once you have diabetes, you (and your doctor) will pay more attention to your health and you may in fact live longer and healthier.

There are a lot of myths and misconceptions about diabetes such as "if you have diabetes, you cannot eat sweets" or "only kids get type 1 diabetes." It is my hope that this book will dispel such myths and misconceptions and that you will come away with the knowledge and skills to take the very best care of your diabetes.

PART ONE

WHAT DOES A DIAGNOSIS OF DIABETES MEAN FOR YOU?

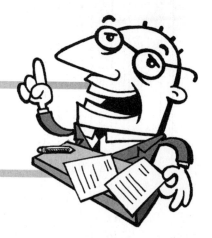

CHAPTER 1

Understanding Diabetes

Diabetes mellitus, or **diabetes**, is an illness in which there is an abnormally high level of **glucose** in the blood. Depending on how high your glucose level is and how long it has been high, you may feel fairly well, or you may be so sick that you require hospitalization. Usually, your doctor will test you for diabetes if you have **symptoms** such as thirst, frequent urination, weight loss, blurred vision, and fatigue. This chapter helps you understand how diabetes is defined and classified and how physicians test for the disease.

Defining Glucose and Its Uses in the Body

Glucose is a sugar and is one of the energy sources of the body. Some organs in our bodies, such as the brain, are particularly dependent upon glucose as an energy source, so it is very important that the body maintain the amount of glucose in the blood in the normal range: if the level is too high or too low, there are serious consequences. To avoid these consequences, the body has a complex set of mechanisms to keep the glucose in the normal range.

The liver is in charge of taking up and releasing glucose into the bloodstream. After a meal, the blood carrying nutrients from digestion first flows through the liver, which removes the excess glucose. When the glucose level in the blood drops (for example, after fasting or exercising), the liver does the opposite and releases glucose into the bloodstream. The liver knows how to regulate the level of glucose in the blood because it receives signals from **hormones**, which are chemical messengers in the blood. The two hormones that are particularly important in diabetes are **insulin** and **glucagon**.

These hormones are produced in the **islets of Langerhans** of the **pancreas**, an elongated organ located behind and below the stomach in the abdomen. There are about a million islets in a normal pancreas, and they consist of several types of cells—the **beta cells** make insulin and the **alpha cells** make glucagon (see Figure 1-1).

In a person with diabetes, the beta cells in the islets fail, and this alters the balance of insulin and glucagon actions on the tissues. The cause and degree of beta cell failure varies in different kinds of diabetes, as described later in this chapter in the section "What Kinds of Diabetes Are There, and Which Kind Do You Have?"

INSULIN

Insulin is the hormone that ensures that the glucose entering the bloodstream from the digestion of food is removed from the blood. It does this by switching the body's **metabolism** so that it uses glucose instead of fat for its energy needs. Insulin also signals the body to make **glycogen** (a storage form of glucose) and to use glucose to make **triglycerides** (another important energy source) for storage in fat

Figure 1-1   Alpha and Beta Cells of the Islets of Langerhans Secrete Glucagon and Insulin

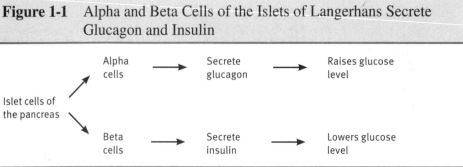

cells. Insulin does all this by its effects on liver cells, muscle cells, and fat cells (see Figure 1-2).

- In the liver, insulin makes the liver cells convert glucose into glycogen, a storage form of glucose, and make triglycerides, a storage form of fat.
- In the muscles, insulin allows the glucose transport into the muscle cells.
- In the fat tissues, insulin stops the breakdown of triglycerides and release of fatty acids into the bloodstream.

GLUCAGON

Glucagon acts in an opposite manner to insulin: it switches the body's metabolism so that it uses fatty acids instead of glucose as its energy source, and it signals the body to increase glucose production. Glucagon achieves this by instructing the liver cells to break down glycogen and release glucose into the bloodstream. It also signals the fat tissues to break down triglycerides and release glycerol and fatty acids into the blood (see Figure 1-3).

Thus, it is the balance of insulin and glucagon that regulates the glucose levels in the blood during the fed and fasting states.

Testing for Diabetes

Your doctor may test you for diabetes if you have symptoms such as thirst, frequent urination, bladder infection, or vaginal yeast infection. Your doctor will measure your blood glucose level, and if it is 200 milligrams per deciliter (mg/dl) or higher,

Figure 1-2   Summary of Effects of Insulin on Liver, Muscle, and Fat Cells

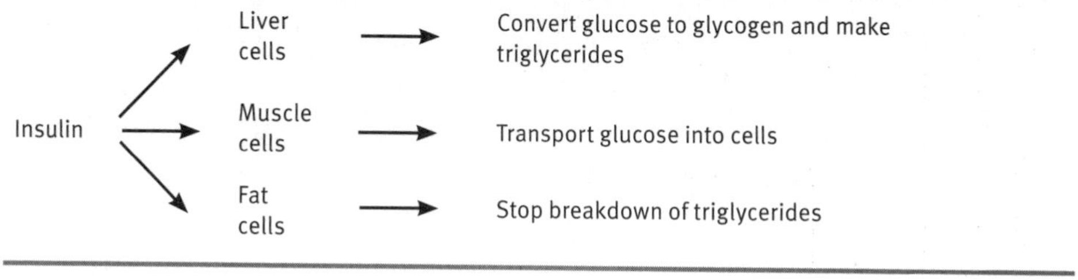

Insulin →

Liver cells → Convert glucose to glycogen and make triglycerides

Muscle cells → Transport glucose into cells

Fat cells → Stop breakdown of triglycerides

Figure 1-3   Summary of Effects of Glucagon on Liver and Fat Cells

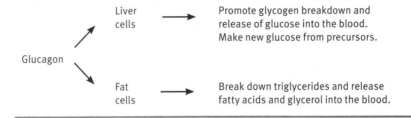

Glucagon → Liver cells → Promote glycogen breakdown and release of glucose into the blood. Make new glucose from precursors.

Glucagon → Fat cells → Break down triglycerides and release fatty acids and glycerol into the blood.

then you have diabetes and no further testing is necessary. If your glucose level is less than 200 mg/dl, then additional tests may be necessary, as described in the next section on screening for diabetes.

Screening for Diabetes

The American Diabetes Association (ADA) has specific guidelines about who should get screened for diabetes, at what age screening should start, and what tests should be used.

- Start screening at the age of forty-five. If the test is normal, repeat every three years.
- Screen adults younger than forty-five if they are overweight and have one or more of the following risk factors:
  - Have a parent, sibling, or child with diabetes
  - Are physically inactive
  - Belong to an ethnic group in which there is higher risk for diabetes (African-American, Latino, Native American, Asian-American, and Pacific Islander)
  - Had diabetes during pregnancy or delivered a baby weighing more than nine pounds
  - Blood pressure readings are 140/90 or higher
  - Have an abnormal lipid profile* with a low level of HDL cholesterol (less than 35 mg/dl) and/or a high level of triglycerides (more than 250 mg/dl)

---

*A **lipid panel or profile** is a blood test for levels of cholesterol, triglycerides, HDL cholesterol, and LDL cholesterol.

- Have a medical condition called **polycystic ovary syndrome (PCOS)**
- Have had previous blood glucose testing that indicated the presence of prediabetes (described later in this chapter)
- Have circulatory problems

There are two screening tests for diabetes, and either is acceptable:

- A fasting glucose level after an overnight fast
- An **oral glucose tolerance test (OGTT)**, in which you drink 75 grams of glucose after an overnight fast and your glucose level is measured two hours later

The ADA recommends that doctors use the fasting glucose test because it is easier to do. If the fasting glucose level is abnormal, but not squarely in the diabetes range, your doctor may go on to do an OGTT.

Table 1-1 is a summary of the tests and the blood glucose levels that determine whether a person has diabetes or prediabetes.

FASTING BLOOD GLUCOSE TEST

The ADA defines fasting glucose levels of less than 100 mg/dl as normal and 126 mg/dl or higher as being in the diabetic range. If fasting glucose level is 126 mg/dl or higher, a confirmatory test is required on another day before a diagnosis of diabetes can be made. A fasting glucose level between 100 and 125 mg/dl is defined as **impaired fasting glucose (IFG)**. This means that you do not yet have diabetes, but are likely to develop diabetes in the future.

Table 1-1 American Diabetes Association Criteria for the Diagnosis of Diabetes		
Clinical Diagnosis	**Fasting Plasma Glucose (FPG) (mg/dl)**	**Oral Glucose Tolerance Test (OGTT) (mg/dl)**
Normal	Less than 100	Less than 140
Impaired fasting glucose (prediabetes)	100–125	—
Impaired glucose tolerance (prediabetes)	—	140–199
Diabetes	126 or above	200 or above

ORAL GLUCOSE TOLERANCE TEST (OGTT)

With the glucose tolerance test, a two-hour glucose value of 200 mg/dl or above is considered to be in the diabetes range and a value below 140 mg/dl is normal. If you have a glucose value between 140 and 200 mg/dl, you have **impaired glucose tolerance (IGT)** and are likely to develop diabetes in the future. You are also at higher risk for developing heart disease.

Because people with IFG and IGT are at higher risk for developing diabetes, the current recommendation is to refer to these patients as having prediabetes.

What Kinds of Diabetes Are There, and Which Kind Do You Have?

There are actually many different kinds of diabetes. All types of diabetes involve inadequate beta cell function, but some also involve problems with the body responding less effectively to insulin (this is known as **insulin resistance**). The ADA has categorized the different kinds of diabetes into four main groups:

- Type 1 diabetes
- Type 2 diabetes
- Other specific types of diabetes
- Gestational diabetes

TYPE 1 DIABETES

In **type 1 diabetes** (formerly referred to as juvenile onset diabetes or **insulin-dependent diabetes mellitus**), a person's immune system attacks its own beta cells and destroys them. This is known as **autoimmune injury**. To control the elevated glucose levels, a person with this kind of diabetes has to be treated with insulin injections. Most people with this kind of diabetes are thin.

TYPE 2 DIABETES

Type 2 diabetes (formerly called adult-onset diabetes or **non-insulin-dependent diabetes mellitus**) is the most common type of diabetes. If you have **type 2 diabetes**, you are **insulin resistant**, which means you need more insulin to lower your blood glucose levels. You also have some beta cell loss in your pancreas, but not to the same extent as in type 1 diabetes. Most of the people with this kind of diabetes are overweight or obese.

OTHER TYPES OF DIABETES

There are less common forms of diabetes in which there is a specific cause for the beta cell failure or problems with insulin function. Some of these conditions are extremely rare, so I discuss only the more common ones in the following sections.

Diabetes Due to Gene Mutations

Maturity onset diabetes of the young (MODY) refers to diabetes that occurs in childhood or adolescence (before age twenty-five) and is inherited in an autosomal dominant fashion; that is, if you have the condition, half of your children are also likely to have it. About one in one hundred people with diabetes have MODY. There are six known genetic defects for this kind of diabetes. One of the genetic defects (called MODY 2) is in the gene that enables the beta cells to sense the body's glucose level (the glucose kinase gene) and so regulate insulin release. MODY 2 is usually easily controlled with oral medications that stimulate insulin release. People with this type of diabetes are usually not obese.

About one in one hundred people with diabetes have a genetic defect in the mitochondria (the energy generating machinery of the cell). The genetic defect seems to cause premature aging of the insulin-secreting beta cells. Since mitochondria are always inherited from the mother and not the father, this is a maternally inherited form of diabetes. The mitochondrial mutation also leads to nerve damage in the ear, so that people with this form of diabetes are frequently deaf.

Diabetes Due to Pancreatic Damage

Because the pancreas is responsible for producing insulin, any damage to the pancreas will cause diabetes. Examples of damage to the pancreas include surgical removal of the pancreas to fight pancreatic cancer and severe pancreatitis (inflammation of the pancreas). Cystic fibrosis may lead to the development of diabetes in early adulthood because of damage to the pancreas and the beta cells.

Two conditions that cause an excess deposition of iron in the pancreas can also damage the beta cells and cause diabetes: hemochromatosis and thalassemia major. In the United States, five in one thousand people carry the genetic defect that causes hemochromatosis. Individuals with this genetic defect absorb more iron than they should, causing pancreatic damage. If you have thalassemia major, you require frequent blood transfusions, and this leads to an iron overload that damages the pancreas.

Diabetes Related to Excessive Hormone Production

There are a number of hormones that oppose the effects of insulin. Examples are cortisol, growth hormone, catecholamines, and glucagon. Tumors that make excess amounts of these hormones can cause diabetes.

Diabetes Induced by Medications

If you have limited beta cell function, using prescription medicines that either decrease insulin effectiveness and/or further decrease beta cell function can cause diabetes. For example, steroids such as prednisone and dexamethasone, which are used to treat inflammation, can cause blood glucose to rise in some people. Niacin, a drug used to lower triglyceride levels and raise HDL cholesterol levels, reduces insulin effectiveness and can cause an increase in blood glucose.

Drugs that are used to suppress the immune system after an organ transplant can cause both insulin resistance and reduced beta cell activity, causing diabetes.

GESTATIONAL DIABETES

Being pregnant increases the body's insulin needs. Diabetes develops when a pregnant woman has limited beta cell capacity and cannot respond to the additional insulin demand. This is referred to as **gestational diabetes**. Often glucose levels become normal after delivery, but anyone who has experienced gestational diabetes has a higher risk of developing type 2 diabetes in the future. There is more information about gestational diabetes in Chapter 13.

Summary

- The level of glucose in the blood is regulated by the balance of two hormones: insulin and glucagon.
- Diabetes occurs when there is a deficiency of the insulin-secreting beta cells. In some kinds of diabetes, the body is also less responsive to the insulin—this condition is known as insulin resistance.
- A diagnosis of diabetes is made if you have symptoms of diabetes and a blood glucose level of 200 mg/dl or more.
- Doctors routinely screen people for diabetes when they reach the age of forty-five. If you have risk factors for diabetes, you may be screened earlier.

- On screening, if your fasting glucose level is 126 mg/dl or more, you have diabetes.

- In type 1 diabetes, the immune system attacks and destroys the beta cells. People with this type of diabetes require insulin injections for survival.

- In type 2 diabetes, there is both beta cell deficiency and insulin resistance. Being overweight or obese increases the risk for type 2 diabetes.

- Gestational diabetes occurs due to the increased insulin demand during pregnancy, and it usually resolves after birth, although the woman is at higher risk for diabetes in the future.

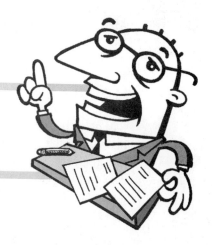

CHAPTER 2

Causes of Diabetes: Genes and Environment

Diabetes occurs as an interaction between the genes that you inherit and the environment in which you live. In type 1 diabetes, we know a fair bit about the genes, but relatively little about how environmental factors impact the disease. In contrast, for type 2 diabetes, the genetic causes are largely unknown, but we know that obesity and lack of exercise are important environmental risk factors.

Type 1 Diabetes

In the United States, there are approximately 1 million people with type 1 diabetes, and about thirty thousand new cases are diagnosed each year. Type 1 diabetes can occur at any age and in any ethnicity, but is more common in children and young adults of Caucasian ancestry. Most cases occur in families where there is no history of type 1 diabetes, but when you have a family member with type 1 diabetes, your risk of getting the disease is higher. Over the past forty years, there has been an increase in the **incidence** of type 1 diabetes in many countries, and it is occurring in younger children. For example, we have good data for Finland: in 1953, the incidence of diabetes was twelve people per one hundred thousand. In 1996, the incidence had increased to forty-five people per one hundred thousand.

WHAT CAUSES TYPE 1 DIABETES?

Type 1 diabetes occurs when the immune system that normally protects the body against infections goes wrong and attacks the beta cells that make insulin. There are genetic factors and environmental factors that cause the immune system to do this.

Type 1 Diabetes and Genetics

Scientists have identified a number of genes that increase an individual's risk for developing type 1 diabetes. The genes that are particularly important include the following:

- **Several genes located in a region of the human genome called human leukocyte antigen (HLA).** Two of the genes (called DR and DQ) code for proteins that help the immune system recognize foreign proteins such as those that make up viruses and bacteria. There are many forms of these two genes, and the ones that increase the individual's susceptibility to type 1 diabetes are called DR3.DQ2 and DR4.DQ8.

- **The insulin gene.** It has been shown that insulin teaches the immune system not to react against the beta cells—this teaching process is referred to as inducing tolerance. People with type 1 diabetes are more likely to have a form of the insulin gene that is less effective in maintaining tolerance.

These genetic factors explain why the risk of type 1 diabetes is increased if you have a family member with the disease. If you have a family member with type 1 diabetes, your risk is 5 to 6 percent, compared to the risk in the general population, which is 0.4 percent. In identical twins this risk increases to 30 to 40 percent. Table 2-1 summarizes the risk if a family member has type 1 diabetes:

Table 2-1   Genetic Risk of Type 1 Diabetes Based on Family History

Family member	Relative risk of getting type 1 diabetes, %
Affected mother	3
Affected father	6
Affected brother or sister	6 to 25*
Affected identical twin	30 to 40

*The risk related to the siblings depends on the inheritance pattern of the susceptible immune genes.

Source: Adapted from Atkinson MA, Maclaren NK. "The pathogenesis of insulin-dependent diabetes mellitus." *N Engl J Med* 1994; 331:1428–36.

DID YOU KNOW?

Beta Cells and Antibodies

When the beta cells are attacked by the immune system, the body produces four types of **antibodies** against the proteins made by the beta cells: glutamic acid decarboxylase (GAD) antibody, islet cell antibody (ICA), ICA 512 antibody, and insulin antibody. Your doctor can measure these **autoantibodies** if there is a question of whether you have type 1 or type 2 diabetes.

Type 1 Diabetes and the Environment

The environment plays a big role in the development of type 1 diabetes—in fact it's twice as important as the genes. The evidence for this comes from several different observations:

- First, for the past forty years, the incidence of type 1 diabetes has been increasing, and it is occurring in younger children. This time period is too short for this to be a change in the genetic makeup of the population.

- Second, type 1 diabetes is more common in the northern latitudes (Scandinavia) and becomes less frequent as you go toward the equator. This is not because people at the equator are genetically protected—when they migrate to northern latitudes, they too become susceptible to type 1 diabetes. For example, it was recently shown that Pakistani children born and raised in England have a higher risk for developing type 1 diabetes compared to children who have lived in Pakistan all their lives.

What is it in the environment that increases the risk of getting type 1 diabetes? We do not know. However, there have been a number of hypotheses: one hypothesis relates type 1 diabetes to infections with viruses such as rubella and Coxsackie B4; another hypothesis relates type 1 diabetes to the consumption of cow's milk. So far, neither of these has been confirmed as being the culprit.

One reason it is hard to figure out which environmental factor is important is that the factor may be important for *initiating* the autoimmune process, but not for maintaining it. Since the immune attack starts many years before a person develops diabetes, it is difficult to figure out what environmental factor was present right at the beginning when the autoimmune process first started. There has been a suggestion that in the developed countries, a lack of childhood infections means that the immune system does not develop properly, and this leads to autoimmunity and the development of conditions such as asthma and diabetes. This theory is known as the hygiene hypothesis.

Other Autoimmune Diseases in People with Type 1 Diabetes

The genetic and environmental factors that increase the risk for type 1 diabetes also increase the risk for other autoimmune diseases. Up to 20 percent of people with type 1 diabetes also have autoimmune thyroid disease, especially underactive thyroid disease (**Hashimoto's thyroiditis**). Once in a while, we also see thyroid overactivity (**Graves' disease**) accompanying type 1 diabetes. Another disease that occurs more frequently in people with type 1 diabetes is **celiac disease**. In this disease, a person is very sensitive to gluten in wheat. About 5 percent of children diagnosed with type 1 diabetes have gluten sensitivity. **Addison's disease**, a rare condition in which there is autoimmune failure of the adrenal glands, also occurs with slightly increased frequency in people with type 1 diabetes.

HOW IS TYPE 1 DIABETES TREATED?

Type 1 diabetes is treated using insulin injections. Oral medicines that are used to treat type 2 diabetes do not work in people with type 1 diabetes because they depend on having the pancreas still making significant amounts of insulin. Early in the disease, a person with type 1 diabetes still has the ability to make and release insulin, and so you will require only a small amount of insulin to keep glucose under control. This early period is referred to at the as the **honeymoon phase** and can last from a few months to several years. Eventually, however, most of the beta cells are lost, and you will be totally dependent on insulin injections for your insulin needs.

Research into Preventing Type 1 Diabetes

Type 1 diabetes occurs because of an autoimmune attack against the beta cells. If we could turn off the immune attack, then we could potentially prevent type 1 diabetes. That this might be possible was suggested by clinical research with drugs that are normally used to prevent rejection of transplanted organs such as kidneys and hearts. When these transplant drugs, which work by suppressing the immune system, were given to patients newly diagnosed with type 1 diabetes, they prolonged the honeymoon phase. The problem, however, was that these drugs had to be given continuously to be effective, and they also have serious side effects such as life-threatening infections and even cancer. For recipients of organ transplants, the benefits of these drugs clearly outweigh the risks, but this is not the case for diabetes. These studies did, however, provide support for this approach to diabetes prevention, and they opened the door for other therapies targeting the immune system.

Currently, a drug called humanized OKT3 is being investigated: in short-term clinical research studies with twelve days of drug, it has been shown to prolong the honeymoon phase in new onset type 1 patients. The drug has a number of advantages: first, it does not have to be given continuously, and second, its side effects appear to be fairly modest. The problem is that the effect is not absolute and permanent—although it slows the beta cells loss, it does not stop it. Additional studies are in progress to see if giving more than one course will be more effective. A number of other immune modulating drugs are also being evaluated to see if they will prolong the honeymoon. Recently, a three-step procedure for eliminating the immune cells that are attacking the beta cells was shown to be successful in prolonging the honeymoon phase. In this procedure, stem cells that can remake some of the cells of the immune system are first collected from the blood of the patient. Then the patient is given chemotherapy to kill off the immune cells that are attacking the beta cells. The third step is to inject the collected stem cells back into the patient to make new immune cells, which presumably will not attack the beta cells. Fifteen people with new onset type 1 diabetes received this treatment, and fourteen of them did not require insulin therapy during the follow-up period of the study, which lasted from 7 to 36 months (average of 18.8 months). It remains to be shown if this beneficial effect is long lasting and whether the procedure is safe in the long term.

Even though the current research studies are being done in people with type 1 diabetes who are in the honeymoon phase, it is expected that if the studies are positive, the therapy will be used in people who are at high risk of developing type 1 diabetes in the future. The National Institutes of Health are funding a consortium called TrialNet to coordinate many of these studies. You can find out more information about these studies at the TrialNet website (diabetestrialnet.org).

Type 2 Diabetes

Type 2 diabetes is the most common form of diabetes in the world. It affects about 17 million people in the United States. In the past, it occurred mostly in middle-aged and older individuals, but nowadays it is often seen in younger people, including children and teenagers. There are more new cases of type 2 diabetes in the United States than ever before, and there are many reasons for this:

- Obesity increases the risk for diabetes, and there has been a dramatic increase in the **prevalence** of obesity (number of people who are obese). The increase in the rate of diabetes parallels the increase in the rate of obesity (see Figure 2-1).
- Diabetes occurs more frequently in older individuals, and the population is aging.
- Ethnic minorities, especially African-Americans, Hispanics, and Asian-Americans, have a higher risk of type 2 diabetes, and there has been an increase in these populations in the United States.
- There is a heightened awareness of diabetes because it has been widely reported in the media in recent years, and so people may be diagnosed earlier than before.
- Recent changes in the way diabetes is diagnosed (measuring fasting glucose rather than doing a two-hour oral glucose tolerance test) have also made it easier to diagnose diabetes.

WHAT CAUSES TYPE 2 DIABETES?

People get type 2 diabetes because

- They are insulin resistant—that is, compared to an **insulin sensitive** person, more insulin is needed to have the same effect (see Chapter 1).
- They have lost beta cells so that they are not able to make enough insulin for the body's needs.

Genetic and environmental factors combine to cause both the insulin resistance and the beta cell loss.

Type 2 Diabetes and Genes

The evidence that genes are important comes from the following observations:

Figure 2-1   Prevalence of Obesity and Diabetes by State in 1994 and 2004

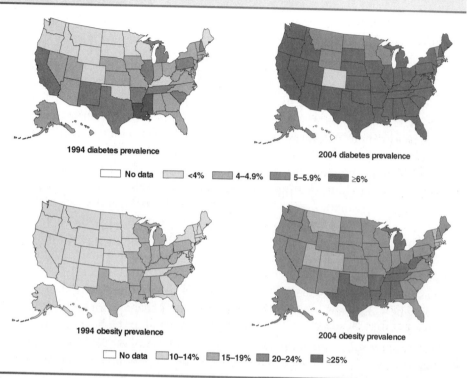

Source: Adapted from data at www.cdc.gov.

- Some ethnic groups are at very high risk for developing diabetes. For example, over 50 percent of the adult Pima Indians living in Arizona have diabetes. People with Caucasian ancestry generally have a lower risk for type 2 diabetes. The risk of diabetes is less in those Pima Indians who also have some European ancestry.

- Type 2 diabetes runs in families. If one parent has type 2 diabetes, the risk that his or her child will develop diabetes in the future is 40 percent, and the risk increases to 70 percent if both parents have diabetes. Also, if you compare identical to nonidentical twins, the risk of a second twin getting diabetes is higher if they are identical.

Sequencing of the human genome has allowed researchers to look for genes that increase the risk of developing type 2 diabetes. Recently, studies of families where multiple members have type 2 diabetes have identified ten regions of the human genome where genetic alterations increase the risk for type 2 diabetes. Interestingly, some of the genetic alterations are in genes that regulate the development or function of the insulin-producing beta cells.

Type 2 Diabetes and Environment

Even though you may have the genetic susceptibility to develop type 2 diabetes, whether you actually get the disease greatly depends on your diet and physical activity. The most important environmental factor for type 2 diabetes is obesity, because having more fat causes insulin resistance. However, not all fat is the same as far as insulin resistance is concerned—fat that is inside the abdomen (visceral fat) is particularly problematic. Women with a waist circumference greater than thirty-five inches (88 cm) and men with a waist circumference greater than forty inches (102 cm) are more likely to have visceral fat and be insulin resistant.

How does visceral fat lead to insulin resistance? We don't know for sure, but scientists have made some interesting observations. People with more visceral fat have higher fatty acid levels in their blood, and this may be important in the development of insulin resistance. We also know that the visceral fat cells release chemicals (such as the hormone adiponectin) that can influence the action of insulin.

As in type 1 diabetes, the beta cell injury in type 2 diabetes starts several years before the development of diabetes. The factors that cause the beta cell injury are not well understood. Visceral fat again may be important, releasing chemical factors that are harmful to the beta cells. Early in the disease process, there are still sufficient beta cells to keep the glucose levels normal. However, in conditions where there is additional need for insulin, the beta cells may not be able to respond adequately and diabetes can develop:

- Gaining weight and not exercising are by far the most common reasons for needing additional insulin.

- Pregnancy increases the need for insulin, and that is why some women get gestational diabetes. After delivery, the insulin needs decline and the diabetes resolves. However, the underlying problem of the injured beta cells does not resolve after delivery, and may even get worse. This means that in future pregnancies the woman will definitely develop diabetes, and may do so even earlier in the pregnancy. Eventually, the beta cell failure progresses so much that even without the additional stress of pregnancy, the glucose levels are elevated and the woman is diagnosed with type 2 diabetes.

- Certain medicines increase insulin needs. For example, steroids (such as prednisone) increase insulin resistance, and when given in large doses for an inflammatory condition such as asthma or rheumatoid arthritis, can cause diabetes in a person with injured beta cells. Usually the diabetes resolves once the steroids are discontinued. Niacin, a drug used to lower triglyceride levels in the blood, when given in very large doses, can also cause insulin resistance, and if a person is susceptible, he or she will get prediabetes (see Chapter 1) or even diabetes. The medicines given after an organ transplant can affect both beta cell function and insulin resistance,

DID YOU KNOW?

Research into Preventing Type 2 Diabetes

There is limited information about why the beta cells fail in people with type 2 diabetes. However, we do know that weight gain and obesity are very important factors in the development of type 2 diabetes. One theory as to why obesity is harmful is that it causes insulin resistance, which increases the workload on the beta cell because more insulin must be produced. Initially the beta cells cope, but eventually this results in beta cell exhaustion and failure. If obesity is reduced or insulin resistance is lowered with medications, then the beta cell failure might not happen, and the development of diabetes could be prevented or delayed. Several large clinical studies have been performed to test this hypothesis.

A study from Sweden, called the Swedish Obesity Surgery Study, looked at the benefits of bariatric surgery on obese individuals over a ten-year period. There was more weight loss and significantly less likelihood (7 percent versus 24 percent) of developing diabetes in the group that had the surgery compared to a nonsurgery control group. There have been a number of other smaller studies that have given the same results.

The Diabetes Prevention Program (DPP) was a randomized clinical trial in 3,234 overweight men and women, aged twenty-five to eighty-five years, who showed impaired glucose tolerance. Results from this study indicated that intervention with a low-fat diet and 150 minutes of moderate exercise per week (equivalent to a brisk thirty-minute walk five times a week) reduces the risk of progression to type 2 diabetes by 58 percent when compared to a matched control group. Another arm of this trial demonstrated that taking 850 mg of the medication metformin twice daily reduced the risk of developing type 2 diabetes by 31 percent, but the medicine was relatively ineffective in people who were either less obese or in the older age group.

Thus, if we could reverse the obesity epidemic in the United States, a substantial decrease in the onset of type 2 diabetes would occur. The prevention of type 2 diabetes is a public health problem in that lifestyle changes are likely to be more effective than treatment with medications. For example, schools can promote physical activity and healthy diets. Cities can ensure that there are sidewalks for people to walk on and that there are bike lanes so that people can safely engage in a more active lifestyle.

and almost 20 percent of people who are taking medicines to prevent rejection of a transplant can develop diabetes. Diabetes may resolve once the transplant medicines are adjusted, and the transplant patient should not stop the immunosuppressant medicines just because of the diabetes.

HOW IS TYPE 2 DIABETES TREATED?

If you are diagnosed with type 2 diabetes, you will be treated for two problems: insulin resistance and impaired insulin release.

The most important thing your doctor will ask you to do, even before prescribing any medicines, is to lose weight by exercising and reducing the calories in your diet. These two things will reduce the insulin resistance significantly. We know that weight loss really works, because when obese patients undergo gastric bypass surgery and reduce the total number of calories they eat, a lot of them (up to 80 percent of patients in some clinical studies) are able to stop their diabetes medicines and their glucose levels became normal.

Your doctor will prescribe medicines if exercise and dietary changes do not control your glucose levels. The medicines work in a variety of ways:

- They slow down glucose absorption from the gut.
- They reduce glucose production from the liver.
- They stimulate insulin release from the remaining beta cells.
- They make the body more responsive to the circulating insulin (decrease insulin resistance).
- They slow stomach emptying and suppress your appetite.

More than one medicine may be necessary to get your glucose levels in the target range. If the oral medicines are not able to adequately control the glucose levels, you are unable to tolerate the side effects, or you have other medical conditions that prevent you taking them, then your doctor will start you on insulin.

During your clinic visit, your doctor will also take into consideration other health issues that are common in people with type 2 diabetes such as high blood pressure and cholesterol problems. If any of these conditions are present, your doctor may give you prescriptions to treat them, as well.

Summary

- Both type 1 and type 2 diabetes occur as a result of interactions between the genes you inherit and environmental factors.

- Type 1 diabetes can occur at any age, but it is more common in children and young adults of Caucasian ancestry. The risk increases if you have a family member with the disease.

- In type 1 diabetes, the genes coding for proteins of the immune system are the most important. Much less is known about the environmental factors.

- People with type 1 diabetes are more prone to other autoimmune diseases such as celiac disease and autoimmune thyroid disease.

- The treatment for type 1 diabetes is insulin replacement using injections or an insulin pump.

- Type 2 diabetes runs in families, but even though you may have inherited the at-risk genes, environmental factors are much more important in determining whether you will develop the condition. Gaining weight (especially around the waist) and lack of exercise are two risk factors for type 2 diabetes.

- Type 2 diabetes is treated with diet, exercise, and medicines.

CHAPTER 3

Complications of Diabetes

One of the problems with diabetes is that the person with the disease usually feels fine and there are no symptoms even when the glucose levels are in the 100 to 200 mg/dl range. Therefore, it is easy to ignore the diabetes. Eventually, there *are* symptoms, but often, they are due to diabetes-related complications. It is therefore important for people with diabetes to understand the consequences of poor glucose control and to make the effort to control the diabetes even when they feel well.

You can think of these consequences as short- and long-term complications. Short-term complications are due to high glucose levels for a period of hours, days, or weeks. Long-term complications are due to elevated glucose levels over a period of years.

Short-Term Complications

The short-term complications that occur in people with diabetes include the following:

- Dehydration
- Weakness and fatigue

- Vaginal or penile yeast infections
- Weight loss
- Blurred vision
- Confusion

The degree of insulin deficiency and the level of blood glucose elevation will determine which of these short-term complications are present. If glucose levels are only slightly elevated, there may not be any symptoms, and diabetes is diagnosed only if the glucose is measured as part of a regular screening.

Glucose does not appear in the urine until the blood glucose level is above 200 mg/dl. When this happens, glucose in the urine can cause bladder or kidney infections (especially in women), vaginal yeast infections, and an infection of the skin of the penis (balanoposthitis). High levels of glucose impair the kidneys' ability to concentrate the urine, and so there is increased urine production and symptoms of frequent urination, thirst, and dehydration. The loss of calories in the urine can cause weight loss, especially if blood glucose levels are very high.

Short-term elevations in glucose can also affect the lens of the eye, causing blurred vision. This is reversible, and the vision returns to normal once the diabetes is treated. Sometimes the blurred vision causes a person to see an ophthalmologist or an optometrist, who then makes the diagnosis of diabetes.

In people who have a severe insulin deficiency (typically people with type 1 diabetes, though it can also occur in type 2 diabetes), a very serious condition called **diabetic ketoacidosis (DKA)** can develop. In DKA, the following symptoms may be present:

- A significant amount of weight loss
- Thirst and frequent urination
- Rapid heart rate
- Nausea and vomiting
- Breathlessness
- Stomach pain
- Severe fatigue
- Blurred vision
- Confusion or coma (if left untreated)

A person who is in DKA has a characteristic appearance: the eyes are sunken, the skin flushed but dry and cool, the tongue is dry, and the breath smells of acetone (like nail polish remover or a room in which apples are kept). The heart rate is fast, and as the illness gets worse, the pulse becomes feeble. Most people are awake, but confusion or coma can occur if the DKA is severe. The urine of a person with DKA has large amounts of glucose and ketones, and there are characteristic abnormalities in the blood tests.

If left untreated, DKA can be life threatening, and people with this condition are usually admitted to the hospital (frequently to the intensive care unit) for treatment with intravenous fluids and insulin.

A significant proportion of people who develop type 1 diabetes first discover their illness when they are in DKA and they get admitted to hospital. Many of these people never get DKA again. Some individuals, however, have another or many episodes of DKA. Infections are an important cause of these repeat DKA episodes. In Chapter 12, you will learn how to manage your diabetes when you are sick and so avoid going into DKA. Failure to take insulin, lack of health-care insurance, and psychological trauma are also risk factors for recurrent DKA.

Sometimes, the insulin deficiency is not severe enough to cause DKA but is still of a sufficient degree to cause very high glucose levels, often 800 mg/dl or more. These very high glucose levels can lead to coma (called a **hyperosmolar coma**). A person in hyperosmolar coma has severe dehydration—the eyes are sunken, the mouth is dry, and the blood pressure is very low. Hyperosmolar coma typically occurs in older individuals, for example, someone living in a nursing home that may not drink enough fluids, but it can also happen in younger individuals who quench their thirst by drinking large amounts of fluids with high sugar content such as juices or regular sodas. Hyperosmolar coma is a very serious medical condition requiring hospital treatment.

Table 3-1 summarizes the main differences in the short-term complications from having elevated glucose levels in people with type 1 and type 2 diabetes. As you can see, some symptoms are more prominent in one or the other, and the symptoms reflect the degree and duration of glucose elevation.

Long-Term Complications

Long-term complications are the effects on the body of prolonged exposure to elevated glucose levels. People with diabetes are understandably fearful of these long-term complications. It is, however, important to emphasize that with good glucose control and treatment of high lipid levels and blood pressure, almost all of these complications can be prevented or their progression arrested. Also, there is a genetic component to complications—even in the presence of poor glucose control, only 40 percent of people with diabetes develop severe complications.

Table 3-1 Differences in Short-Term Complications in Type 1 and Type 2 Diabetes

	Type 1 Diabetes	Type 2 Diabetes
No symptoms (feels fine)	unlikely	common
Thirst and urination, including waking up at night	common	less common
Weakness and fatigue	common	less common
Vaginal or penile yeast infections	less common	common
Eating a lot but losing weight	common	unlikely
Blurred vision	less common	common
DKA	common	less common
Hyperosmolar coma	unlikely	common

DID YOU KNOW?

How Do Glucose Levels Harm Cells?

Exactly how high glucose levels cause harm to the cells of the body is not known. One theory is that the elevated glucose levels deplete **antioxidants** in cells. The chemical reactions in the cells cause the release of **reactive oxygen species** that are neutralized by antioxidants. A deficiency of antioxidants can allow the reactive oxygen species to damage proteins and interfere with chemical reactions of the cells. The obvious question to ask is, What if we take in a lot of antioxidants in our diet—will this prevent the cell injury? A lot of research is currently being done to try to answer this question, but it is too soon to tell if this approach will work.

Long-term complications are categorized into two types: microvascular and macrovascular. This division does not mean that one gets only one or the other—many times people have a little bit of both.

- **Microvascular complications** relate to the small blood vessels and capillaries and lead to kidney, eye, and nerve disease. In people with type 1 diabetes, where the problem is principally of glucose control, microvascular complications are initially more prominent, but once these develop, or with long duration of diabetes, macrovascular complications may also occur.

• **Macrovascular complications** relate to disease of medium-sized and large blood vessels and lead to heart attacks, circulation problems in the legs, and strokes. Generally speaking, people with type 2 diabetes are more prone to the macrovascular complications, because in addition to having elevated glucose values, they often have high blood pressure (**hypertension**), high cholesterol and triglycerides, and low HDL cholesterol. They may develop microvascular disease with time if their glucose levels remain elevated.

Another point to remember is that some of the complications that are seen in people with diabetes (for example cataracts, glaucoma, heart disease) also occur in the absence of diabetes. The difference is that these complications are more frequent in people with diabetes.

DIABETIC EYE DISEASE

Diabetic eye disease includes three conditions: diabetic **retinopathy**, **cataracts**, and **glaucoma**.

Diabetic Retinopathy

At the back of the eye on the **retina** are tiny blood vessels that nourish the nerves of the eye. High glucose levels or high blood pressure can injure the cells lining these blood vessels (retinopathy). The earliest visible abnormalities are pinhead red dots next to the blood vessels that may come and go—these are called microaneurysms or dot hemorrhages. Further injury then causes leakage of blood and fluid into the surrounding areas. The hemorrhages have a characteristic appearance—they are known as blot and flame hemorrhages. The fluid leakage causes yellow deposits called hard exudates. These changes in the back of the eye (also called background retinopathy) do not cause any problems with the vision and the patient is unaware of them. They are, however, of concern because if action is not taken to improve the glucose control and lower the blood pressure, they may progress to more serious injury and vision loss.

If there is progression, the injured blood vessels get blocked and the areas of the retina supplied by these vessels become starved of nutrients. The retina responds by releasing chemicals, such as vascular endothelium growth factor (VEGF), that promote the growth of new blood vessels. This abnormality is called proliferative retinopathy. Unfortunately, these new blood vessels are fragile and can bleed easily. The hemorrhages from these new vessels can cause sudden loss of vision. The hemorrhages and growth factors can also cause scar tissue to develop at the back of the eye. This scar tissue can pull on the retina, causing a **retinal detachment** and vision loss.

The injured blood vessels can also leak fluid and cause swelling in an area of the retina called the macula—this condition, called **macular edema**, can cause the loss of central vision, making it difficult to read or drive.

One way of protecting vision is to use lasers to destroy the parts of the retina that do not have adequate nutrition so that the new blood vessels that are prone to bleeding do not grow. Laser therapy is also used to treat macular edema by removing the areas with very leaky blood vessels. The disadvantage of laser therapy is that it does destroy part of the retina. People who have had extensive laser therapy frequently complain of difficulty with night vision.

Recently, it has been shown that injecting the anticancer drug bevacizumab (Avastin) into the eye can stop the growth of the new blood vessels due to diabetic eye disease. Bevacizumab works by blocking the action of VEGF.

Cataracts

A cataract is a clouding of the lens of the eye so that the person cannot see clearly. The symptoms of cataracts are

- Gradual blurring of the vision
- Glare in bright light or sunlight
- Poor color vision with fading or yellowing of colors
- Double or multiple images when one eye is closed

Cataracts occur as part of the natural aging process, but they occur earlier and more often in people with diabetes. It is thought that the high glucose level causes changes in the proteins inside the cells of the lens, altering the optical properties of the lens. The treatment for cataracts is surgery—the cloudy lens is removed and replaced with an artificial lens.

Glaucoma

The inside of the eye is filled with fluid. New fluid is constantly being made, and the fluid that is being replaced leaves the eye by entering a drainage meshwork toward the front of the eye. Blockage of the drainage system can lead to increased fluid pressure within the eye—a condition called glaucoma. This pressure increase can damage the nerves going from the back of the eye to the brain and cause vision loss. Like cataracts, glaucoma occurs more frequently in people with diabetes.

Glaucoma is treated with eyedrops:

- **Beta-blocker eyedrops** such as timolol (Timoptic), levobunolol (Betagan), and betaxolol (Betoptic) reduce the amount of fluid made. They are usually quite safe, but they can cause breathing problems in patients with asthma or chronic bronchitis.

- **Miotic eyedrops** such as pilocarpine (Isopto Carpine) and carbachol (Isopto Carbachol) contract the iris, opening the drainage channels for the fluid to drain. These drops make the pupil smaller, and initially patients may complain of headache and eyestrain, but both usually get better with time.

- **Carbonic anhydrase inhibitors** such as dorzolamide (Trusopt) also reduce the amount of fluid made. Sometimes people complain of nausea when they use this type of eyedrop.

If the drops do not work, an eye operation to allow the fluid to drain (trabeculectomy) is performed.

Rarely, glaucoma can occur in people with diabetes when there is blood vessel growth in the iris blocking the fluid drainage channels (a condition called iridis rubeosis). This type of glaucoma is usually treated with lasers. It has recently been reported that bevacizumab might also be effective.

DIABETIC KIDNEY DISEASE

The kidneys function to remove excess salt and water and the waste chemicals made by the body. They work a little bit like a strainer—allowing salt, water, small proteins, and various chemicals (but not the large proteins and blood cells) to pass through into the kidney tubules. Later, many of these filtered chemicals as well as small proteins, salt, and water that the body still needs are reabsorbed by the kidney tubules, leaving behind the excess salt, water, and waste chemicals to form the urine.

Over many years, high glucose levels can injure the kidneys' filtering mechanisms as well as the absorption mechanisms. The degree of injury can be assessed with two measurements:

- A **protein** called albumin in the urine
- A chemical called **creatinine** in the blood

Normally, the amount of albumin in the first morning sample of urine is less than 30 mg per gram creatinine, but with kidney damage due to diabetes, this value can increase. When the value is in the 30 to 300 range, it is called **microalbuminuria,** and when it is more than 300, then the condition is called **macroalbuminuria**. Table 3-2 gives the classification of kidney function using urinary albumin measurements.

Creatinine, on the other hand, is a chemical in the bloodstream that is released by muscles and removed from the body by the kidneys. The kidneys are quite efficient at removing the creatinine, and the blood creatinine level does not go up until the kidney damage is significant.

Table 3-2 Classification of Kidney Function Using Urinary Albumin Measurements	
Kidney Function	**Amount of Albumin in First Morning Urine Sample (mg/gram creatinine)**
Normal	Less than 30
Early kidney failure: microalbuminuria	30–300
Severe kidney failure: macroalbuminuria	More than 300

DID YOU KNOW?

Treating High Blood Pressure Helps the Kidneys

Medicines that reduce blood pressure stop the kidney damage from getting worse. Usually your doctor will first prescribe a medicine called **angiotensin converting enzyme (ACE) inhibitor**. The side effects of ACE inhibitors include an increase in the potassium and creatinine levels in the blood, occasionally a cough, and, rarely, facial swelling. The rise in potassium can usually be managed by taking a **diuretic** such as hydrochlorothiazide (HCTZ), a medicine that makes you urinate more, and by avoiding foods high in potassium. Stopping the medicine gets rid of the cough, and your doctor then may switch you to another group of medicines called **angiotensin receptor blockers (ARBs)**, which have the same beneficial effect on diabetic kidney disease as ACE inhibitors. Quite often, ACE inhibitors and ARBs are prescribed together. If these two medicines are insufficient, additional blood pressure medicines are prescribed. Table 3-3 is a list of blood pressure medicines that your doctor may use to treat diabetic kidney disease.

Table 3-3   Medicines for the Treatment of High Blood Pressure

Name of Medicine	Examples (Generic and Trade Names)	How They Work to Lower Blood Pressure
Angiotensin converting enzyme (ACE) inhibitors	Captopril (Capoten) Enalapril (Vasotec) Benazepril (Lotensin) Lisinopril (Prinivil, Zestril) Quinapril (Accupril) Ramipril (Altace) Trandolapril (Mavik)	Work on the renin-angiotensin system
Angiotensin receptor blockers (ARBs)	Losartan (Cozaar) Valsartan (Diovan) Olmesartan (Benicar) Irbesartan (Avapro) Candesartan (Atacand) Telmisartan (Micardis)	Work on the renin-angiotensin system
Beta-blockers	Metoprolol (Lopressor) Atenolol (Tenormin) Carvedilol (Coreg)	Work on blood vessel walls, blocking the action of the sympathetic nervous system, reducing blood pressure
Diuretics	Hydrochlorothiazide (HCTZ) Furosemide (Lasix)	Reduce blood pressure by increasing the amount of salt and water removed by the kidneys
Calcium channel blockers	Amlodipine (Norvasc) Nifedipine (Adalat, Procardia) Diltiazem (Cardizem)	Work on the smooth muscles of the blood vessels, making them relax and so reducing blood pressure
Alpha blockers	Doxazosin (Cardura) Terazosin (Hytrin)	Work on the blood vessel walls, causing the blood vessels to dilate and therefore reducing blood pressure
Central alpha agonist	Clonidine (Catapres)	Works in the central nervous system, inhibiting the sympathetic system

Treatment of diabetic kidney disease is directed at preventing further damage to the kidneys with the following interventions:

- Maintain good glucose control.
- Control blood pressure.
- Restrict protein intake: there is some evidence that kidney disease is made worse by a diet that is high in protein, so your doctor may recommend a low-protein diet.
- Stop smoking.
- Reduce weight: obesity is a risk factor for microalbuminuria, and it is possible that weight loss can reduce the protein loss.
- Avoid medications that can cause further kidney damage. (See sidebar, "Being Careful with the Kidneys.")

In severe kidney failure, when 80 to 90 percent of kidney function is lost, the kidneys can no longer remove the waste products and excess salt and water from the body. When this happens, the person with kidney failure will need **dialysis**, a medical procedure for removing toxic waste products from the blood, and/or a kidney transplant. Additional information on dialysis and kidney transplantation is available at the National Kidney Foundation website (see Resources).

DIABETIC NERVE DISEASE

If you have elevated blood glucose for a long time, many different nerves in your body can get damaged—a condition known as **neuropathy**. In the following sec-

---

DID YOU KNOW?

Being Careful with the Kidneys

Kidneys with early diabetes changes are particularly sensitive to injury from medicines such as nonsteroidal anti-inflammatories, which include ibuprofen (Advil, Motrin), naproxen (Naprosyn), indomethacin (Indocin), and others. Although occasional use of these medicines might be fine, you should not take them daily. Talk to your physician about other pain treatments. Contrast media used in x-ray studies can also damage the kidneys, and if you need to have such a procedure, your doctor may prescribe extra fluids, a medicine called N-acetylcysteine, or a sodium bicarbonate infusion to prevent or limit further kidney damage.

tions, I discuss these injuries in terms of the part of the body that is affected and the treatment approach.

Nerve Injury to the Feet

The most common type of nervous system injury in diabetes is to the nerves that innervate the muscles of the feet and transmit sensory information from the feet to the spinal cord. Feet, rather than hands, are affected first because the nerves to the feet are longer. Usually the symptoms start at the toes and gradually go up the foot and leg to the knee (known as stocking distribution). Early on, the injury may present with occasional tingling or slight electrical shocks. As it progresses, the symptoms may get worse with more persistent tingling or burning sensation or feeling cold. With even further damage, the burning and uncomfortable sensation gets better, but then there may be more numbness. Early on, the numbness might be quite mild, but later on the numbness may be so profound that pain cannot be felt. It is this severe form of nerve injury that is of most concern, because a person with this condition may not be aware of the foot injury.

Paralysis of the small muscles of the foot due to diabetic nerve injury can alter the shape of the foot with clawing of the toes and flattening of the arches. When this happens, calluses can develop over pressure points, and then the pressure from the calluses causes ulcers in the tissue underneath.

There are a variety of treatments for pain due to neuropathy, and finding the best treatment is really a matter of trying them out. Good glucose control is important because the pain is worse with poor control. Simple things such as acetaminophen (Tylenol) at night might be sufficient. Your doctor may also prescribe tricyclic antidepressants such as amitriptyline (Elavil) taken one to two hours before bedtime to help the pain. Amitriptyline causes drowsiness, and this can be a good thing for a good night's sleep. Sometimes, however, the sleepiness extends into the day, in which case your doctor may ask you to try another tricyclic antidepressant that causes less drowsiness. Other side effects that can occur include dry eyes and dry mouth, constipation, and difficulty urinating. If these side effects cannot be tolerated, then one of the newer anticonvulsants, gabapentin (Neurontin), can be used. The common side effects of gabapentin are drowsiness, fatigue, and imbalance. Recently, a medicine related to gabapentin, called pregabalin (Lyrica), was approved for painful neuropathy. There is no evidence that it is any better than gabapentin. Duloxetine (Cymbalta) is another antidepressant that is also useful in treating neuropathy.

Capsaicin, a chemical found in hot peppers, can be used to treat the pain from diabetic neuropathy. The capsaicin cream Zostrix (available over the counter) is rubbed on the painful areas of the feet two to four times a day. Initially the burning feels worse and there may be redness, but if you persist, the burning gets much better by about the second week. You do have to wash your hands carefully after using it (or use gloves), otherwise you may end up with burning eyes or face.

For a very small number of people, none of these treatments are sufficient to control the pain, and it may be necessary to take stronger pain medicines such as tramadol (Ultram) or morphine, preferably under the supervision of physicians at a pain control clinic.

Foot ulcers occur in about 5 percent of people with diabetes. It is important to emphasize that foot ulcers can almost always be prevented, and there are many people with neuropathy and circulation problems of their feet who never get foot ulcers.

People with diabetes are at higher risk for foot ulcers for the following reasons:

- Diabetic nerve injury changes the shape of the foot and leads to callus formation at pressure points.

- Diabetic nerve injury impairs sensation, and you may be unaware of injury. For example, you may step on something sharp and not realize it.

- Nerve injury to the sweat glands in the feet can lead to dry feet and cracks in skin.

- Damage to the small blood vessels causes swelling of the feet.

- Damage to the large blood vessels reduces blood flow to the foot and impairs healing.

So, how can foot ulcers be prevented if some or all of these abnormalities are present?

First, if you have evidence of diabetic neuropathy or foot circulatory problems, see a podiatrist who has an interest in treating diabetic feet. The podiatrist can

- Trim the calluses and reduce the pressure on the underlying tissues

- Prescribe custom orthotics that spread the foot pressures and so prevent the development of new calluses

- Treat fungal infection if present and recommend moisturizing creams for dry skin

- Prescribe custom, extra-depth shoes if the shape of your foot is altered so that it cannot fit into a normal shoe

- Counsel on proper foot care

Second, it is important not to walk barefoot when there is severe numbness. Socks and shoes should be worn at all times. Examine the inside of your shoes regularly (at least daily) to make sure that there are no pebbles, grit, or other objects in the shoes.

Third, examine your feet daily for cuts, swelling, and blisters. Toenails should be cut straight across to avoid the problem of ingrowing toenails.

Fourth, new shoes should be comfortable and well fitting and initially worn only a few hours at a time.

Fifth, if severe foot deformity and numbness is present, then non-weight-bearing exercise, such as riding a stationary bicycle, may be better than weight-bearing exercises such as walking and jogging.

If a blister or foot ulcer develops, it is important to seek medical attention immediately. Depending on the cause, treatments include removal of calluses and dead skin, antibiotics, limiting walking, and treating circulatory problems.

Nerve Injury to the Hands

The same kind of neuropathy that happens in the feet can happen in the hands, but it is less common. Instead, what occurs more often is pinching of the nerves to the hands as they pass through the narrow canals at the elbow and wrist. When this occurs, there is pain and tingling in the fingers of the hand and/or the arm. In **carpal tunnel syndrome**, the median nerve gets pinched in the canal at the wrist. When the ulnar nerve gets pinched at the elbow it is called ulnar nerve entrapment. Both of these conditions occur in the absence of diabetes—for example, carpal tunnel syndrome is a repetitive strain injury. Nerve conduction tests performed by neurologists can help identify carpal tunnel syndrome and ulnar nerve entrapment. The conditions are treated with splints, anti-inflammatory medicines, steroid injections, or surgery.

Injuries to the Nerves of the Face and Eye Muscles

Occasionally, an older person with diabetes will suddenly develop double vision and/or a drooping eyelid. This occurs because one of the three nerves that control the muscles of the eye gets injured. Usually the nerve recovers after a few weeks and the symptoms improve. Similarly, in a condition called **Bell's palsy**, there is paralysis of the facial nerve (seventh cranial nerve), which supplies muscles of the face on one side or the other. Usually, the palsy gets better in a few weeks or months. There is one caveat—since both double vision and the Bell's palsy can occur with other neurological disorders as well, you cannot assume that they are due to diabetes, and they should be evaluated by a specialist when they occur.

Occasionally a person with diabetes will get an injury to the nerve supplying the sweat glands in the face. When this occurs, there is sweating of the face on eating. This condition is referred to as gustatory sweating, and one of the treatments for it is the blood pressure medicine clonidine (Catapres). Sometimes the sweating tends to happen with specific foods such as cheese.

Injury to the Nerves of the Stomach

Longstanding diabetes can also affect the nerves that control stomach emptying and bowel function. If the nerves to the stomach are affected, stomach emptying may be delayed, causing a bloated feeling after eating. If the condition is severe, there may be vomiting of undigested food after many hours. This condition is called **gastroparesis**. Normally, insulin is injected before a meal so that the peak level of the insulin matches the glucose rise after a meal. If gastroparesis is present, however, the glucose rise might be delayed—the resultant mismatch between the insulin peak and the glucose peak can cause low-glucose reactions. The gastroparesis can be intermittent and may be triggered by particular foods, for example, high-fat, high-protein foods. High glucose levels themselves can also worsen the symptoms of gastroparesis.

Gastroparesis is suspected if there is complaint of bloating, vomiting old food, and low-glucose reactions shortly after eating. Sometimes the symptoms are so consistent with the diagnosis that no further testing is necessary. If the diagnosis is uncertain, a test called radioisotope labeled solid food emptying is performed. In this test, an egg sandwich containing a radioactive marker is eaten and a scanner looks at the speed with which the radioactivity leaves the stomach. You can treat gastroparesis by

- Keeping the blood glucose levels stable
- Avoiding high-fat, high-protein foods and choosing low-fat, high-fiber foods instead
- Altering the timing of the insulin injection or the oral diabetes medicines to minimize the risk of low-glucose reactions
- Taking medicines that improve gastric emptying: Metoclopramide (Reglan) works best if it is taken regularly three or four times a day. Side effects include anxiety and drowsiness. Sometimes, people taking metoclopramide get involuntary tics of the facial muscles (called a dystonic reaction), which go away once the medicine is stopped. If this happens, it should not be used again. Erythromycin is an antibiotic that can help stomach emptying and is given before meals. One of the problems with gastroparesis is that the gastric outlet (pylorus) does not relax properly. It has been reported that botulinum toxin (the treatment, called Botox, more popularly known to help wrinkles) injected into the pylorus can help the gastroparesis, but this is still experimental.
- Using an electric gastric stimulator to aid gastric emptying if all the preceding treatments fail

Nerve injury to the bowel can cause intermittent constipation, and over-the-counter laxatives may be used. Sometimes the constipation can alternate with diarrhea, and some individuals can have mostly diarrhea with frequent liquid stools. This can be treated with antidiarrhea medicines such as diphenoxylate with atropine (Lomotil) or loperamide (Imodium). Rarely the diarrhea can be severe and an injectable medicine called octreotide (Sandostatin) might help.

Injury to Nerves to the Bladder and the Penis

When the bladder nerves are affected by prolonged high glucose levels, the bladder may not empty properly, and this can cause urinary incontinence and bladder infections. The problem can be due to either decreased or increased bladder muscle activity. Often an evaluation by a urologist is necessary. If the bladder tends to contract and empty more frequently (overactive bladder), antispasmodic medicines such as oxybutynin (Ditropan) and tolterodine (Detrol) can be helpful. If the problem is inadequate bladder muscle contraction, then a medicine called bethanechol (Urecholine), which stimulates bladder muscles, may help.

Injury to the nerves to the penis can cause an inability to get an adequate erection, called **erectile dysfunction**, which is described in the section "Diabetes and Erectile Dysfunction" later in this chapter.

Injury to the Nerves Supplying the Heart and Blood Vessels

The vagus nerve regulates the heart rate, and when it gets injured due to high blood glucose levels the heart rate is fast even at rest. The fast heart rate by itself is not necessarily harmful, unless the person also has **coronary artery disease**. In this case, the neuropathy can increase the risk of serious heart rhythm problems and even death. Therefore, people with diabetes who have **autonomic neuropathy** affecting the heart should be evaluated by a cardiologist to determine the extent of heart disease.

The nerves to the heart and blood vessels regulate the blood pressure changes that occur when getting up from a lying down position to sitting to standing. If these nerves are injured, you can get light-headed on sitting up or on standing. This is because the blood pressure falls (referred to as **postural hypotension**). It is a condition that can be quite difficult to treat satisfactorily. The following interventions may help:

- Avoid getting dehydrated and increase fluid and salt intake.
- Avoid lying completely flat and sleep either with the head of the bed raised or in a sitting position. This reduces the blood pressure changes with posture.

- Wear support stockings to reduce the blood pooling in the legs.
- Take fludrocortisone (Florinef), a medicine that causes salt retention. The problem is that although the drug helps raise blood pressure when sitting or standing, it can also lead to high blood pressure when lying down, which is not such a good thing.
- Take midodrine (ProAmatine), a newer treatment that constricts the blood vessels and raises blood pressure—your doctor may prescribe this if the other treatments are not effective.

Nerve Injuries in the Leg

Foot drop—that is, paralysis of the muscles that lift the foot at the ankle—occurs from time to time in people with diabetes. It is due to an injury to a nerve called the peroneal nerve. A person with this condition has to lift the affected leg higher than usual when walking. Many times it improves, but sometimes it is permanent, and then it is treated with a leg splint.

There is also a rare condition called **diabetic amyotrophy**, where the injury is to one of the nerves supplying the muscles of the thigh (femoral nerve) and causes severe pain and weakness in the thigh. With good glucose and pain control the symptoms get better over a period of twelve to eighteen months.

Occasionally, a person with diabetic peripheral neuropathy has problems sensing the position of a joint (that is, a deficiency in **proprioception**). This can put significant stresses on ankle or foot joints leading to fractures and joint dislocation. The person will complain of sudden pain and swelling of the foot or ankle, often after a minor foot injury (such as tripping on a curb). This condition is called **Charcot's arthropathy**. The doctor will treat this using a non-weight-bearing leg cast. Medicines called bisphosphonates, such as pamidronate and alendronate (Fosamax), that are usually used to treat osteoporosis can also help.

DIABETES AND OTHER PROBLEMS WITH THE HANDS, FEET, AND JOINTS

The connective tissue in the hands and around joints can be affected by diabetes, especially after many years of the disease. In the hands and feet there is a layer of collagen (fascia) under the skin. Thickening of this fascia in the hands leads to a condition called **Dupuytren's contractures**, causing an inability to straighten fingers, and also a condition called **trigger finger**. When the condition gets severe, surgery may be necessary. Dupuytren's contractures occur in the absence of diabetes, but it is about five times as common in people with diabetes. An inflammation of the fascia in the foot can lead to a condition called **plantar fasciitis**, causing heel pain severe enough to prevent walking. Treatment includes stretching exercises and a night splint, orthotics, physical therapy, and nonsteroidal anti-inflammatory drugs. If these do not work, steroid injections can be tried.

The connective tissue around the joints can also be affected, leading to a decrease in joint flexibility, usually seen in hand, shoulder, and hip joints. People with diabetes are also at risk for **frozen shoulder**—a condition where there is pain, stiffness, and loss of movement at the shoulder joint. Treatment is pain control and physical therapy—it usually gets better, but it may take a year or so.

DIABETES AND PROBLEMS WITH SKIN AND NAILS

There are a number of skin and nail problems that are more commonly seen in people with diabetes. These include the following:

- Fungal infections of the skin (athlete's foot) and nails (**onychomycosis**), which require treatment with antifungal medicines.

- **Acanthosis nigricans**, a darkening of the skin at the back of the neck and under the armpit. The skin has a velvety feel. This condition occurs in people with type 2 diabetes who are very insulin resistant. It does not require any treatment.

- **Necrobiosis lipoidica diabeticorum.** This is seen mostly in people with type 1 diabetes. There is a thinning of the skin on the shins with a reddish yellowish discoloration. Sometimes it can be ulcerated in the middle. Treatment is usually with steroid injections or creams.

- **Lipohypertrophy**, a localized swelling, is caused by repeated insulin injections in one spot. Insulin absorption becomes more erratic in these areas. Stopping injections of insulin in the affected area usually leads to recovery.

- **Shin spots**, or diabetic dermopathy, are brown, oval patches on the shins (and sometimes on the forearms) of people with diabetes. Men are more prone to this than women. There is no treatment for it.

- **Scleredema diabeticorum**, a firm swelling and thickening of the skin of the shoulders and upper back. This condition can be itchy. Treatments include steroid ointment and a medicine called methotrexate.

DIABETES AND CIRCULATORY PROBLEMS

People with diabetes, especially those with type 2 diabetes, are two to five times more likely to have problems with circulation to the heart, the legs, and the head when compared to individuals without diabetes. This is because diabetes predisposes a person to a condition called **atherosclerosis**. If you imagine a blood vessel as a water or drainage pipe, then atherosclerosis is buildup in the pipe narrowing the channel and impairing the flow. In the case of the blood vessel the buildup, called plaque, consists of a core of inflammatory cells, cholesterol, and lipids with a fibrous cap of smooth muscle cells (see Figure 3-1). The plaque can narrow the blood vessel, impairing blood flow. Occasionally the fibrous cap can rupture, and when this happens a blood clot forms, causing an acute blockage of the blood vessel. If the acute blockage happens in one of the blood vessels to the heart, it results in a heart attack. If it occurs in one of the blood vessels supplying brain tissue, it results in a stroke.

What is it about diabetes that predisposes a person to atherosclerosis? First, having high glucose levels for long periods can injure the cells lining the blood vessels, initiating the plaque buildup. Second, the high blood pressure and the elevated lipids frequently present in people with diabetes are known risk factors for plaque buildup. There are also other less well understood factors such as blood clotting factors and platelet function that are also altered in people with diabetes.

Even though people with type 1 diabetes generally do not have high blood pressure and high cholesterol problems, they can develop heart disease after many years. This is especially likely to occur if they have diabetic kidney disease.

Figure 3-1   Artery Containing Plaque Buildup

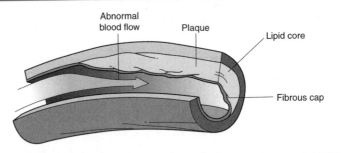

Source: www.nhlbi.nih.gov/health/dci/diseases/cad/cad_causes.html.

Diabetes and the Heart

Diabetes affects the heart in a number of different ways. Atherosclerosis of the coronary arteries (coronary artery disease) can limit the delivery of nutrients to the heart muscle. When this occurs you can develop chest pain with exercise (**angina**). If there is acute blockage then this is referred to as a **heart attack** or **myocardial infarction**.

Heart failure is more common in people with diabetes. Many times it occurs because of heart muscle damage following a heart attack. Long-standing high blood pressure associated with diabetes is also an important cause. It is now also recognized that high glucose levels themselves damage the heart muscles. People with heart failure feel tired, short of breath at rest and/ or on exertion, and have leg swelling.

It is therefore important to have a physical checkup to rule out heart disease before you begin an exercise program. See Chapter 9 for more on exercising with diabetes.

Diabetes and Brain Circulation

Interruptions of blood supply to the brain due to atherosclerosis can lead to transient or permanent neurological abnormalities—referred to as a **transient ischemic attack (TIA)** or **stroke**. Older people with diabetes have an increased risk of memory problems, and it is thought that in at least some of them, this is a result of small strokes.

Diabetes and Circulation to the Legs

When there is atherosclerosis in the blood vessels supplying the leg, the decrease in the blood flow can lead to cramps and pain (typically in the calves) when exercising. This is called **intermittent claudication**, and the pain is relieved by rest. If the blood supply is severely impaired, there is pain even at rest. Eventually, the lack of blood flow can cause tissue death, especially of the toes (**gangrene**). Cigarette smokers are particularly at risk.

Prevention of Circulatory Problems

Circulatory problems, especially heart disease, are the major cause of premature death in people with diabetes, and prevention of these problems is a central goal in the treatment of diabetes. You can take a number of steps to reduce your risk of heart disease and circulatory problems:

- **Improve glucose control.** The target levels are described in Chapter 5.

- **Lower blood pressure.** I have already discussed in the "Diabetic Kidney Disease" section earlier in this chapter the importance of controlling blood pressure. The treatment goal is to get the systolic blood pressure (top number) below 130 mm Hg and the diastolic blood pressure (bottom number) below 80.

- **Take aspirin.** Clinical studies show that aspirin reduces the risk of heart attacks and stroke. Aspirin works by making platelets (the cells in the blood that are responsible for blood clotting) less sticky. Recent studies indicate that lower doses are just as effective as higher doses, so low-dose aspirin therapy (a 75–81 mg dose once a day) is recommended if you already have heart disease or circulatory problems. If you cannot tolerate aspirin because of allergic reaction or another reason, your doctor may prescribe a medicine called clopidogrel (Plavix), which also makes the platelets less sticky. Individuals with type 1 and 2 diabetes without heart disease or circulatory problems should also take low-dose aspirin therapy if they have a strong family history of heart disease; if they have kidney damage, high blood pressure, or lipid problems; if they are smokers; or if they are older than forty years.

- **Stop smoking.** Smoking increases the risk of both macrovascular and microvascular damage in people with diabetes.

- **Improve your lipid profile.** People with type 2 diabetes frequently have abnormalities of their lipid profile—a collective term for cholesterol, triglycerides, HDL cholesterol, and LDL cholesterol levels. Almost all people with type 2 diabetes and many with type 1 diabetes need to take medicines for the lipid abnormalities.

DID YOU KNOW?

Children and Aspirin

Individuals younger than twenty-one years should not take aspirin, because if they are taking it and they get influenza, they are at higher risk of developing a very serious illness called Reye's syndrome. If you are under twenty-one years of age, you should consult your doctor before taking aspirin.

DID YOU KNOW?

The Function of Cholesterol

Cholesterol is an important molecule in the structure of cell membranes and nerve sheaths and is a building block for a number of important hormones. The body absorbs cholesterol from the food we eat, and it also makes new cholesterol in the liver.

Triglycerides are an energy source of the body made in the intestine and the liver. They consist of three fatty acid chains combined with glycerol. Cholesterol and triglycerides combine with proteins to form **lipoprotein particles** that circulate in the blood. These particles include the following:

- **Chylomicrons**
- **Very low-density lipoproteins (VLDL)**
- **Low-density lipoproteins (LDL),** which deliver cholesterol to all the cells in the body
- **High-density lipoproteins (HDL),** which are made in the liver and intestines— HDL cholesterol is known as the good cholesterol

In people with diabetes, the levels of triglycerides are frequently too high and the levels of HDL are too low. In addition, people with diabetes tend to have a form of LDL particles called small, dense LDL, which can abnormally collect in the blood vessel walls and cause atherosclerosis. Research has shown that correcting these lipid abnormalities in people with diabetes reduces the development of atherosclerosis. The goals of treatment are to

- Lower the LDL cholesterol to at least below 100 mg/dl but ideally to 60 to 70 mg/dl
- Lower the triglyceride level to below 150 mg/dl
- Raise the HDL cholesterol to more than 40 mg/dl in men, and to more than 50 mg/dl in women

There are a number of lipid-lowering medicines that a doctor may prescribe. These are summarized in Table 3-4.

Table 3-4 Lipid-Lowering Medicines

Name of Medicine	Examples (Generic and Trade Names)	How It Affects the Lipid Profiles
HMG-CoA reductase inhibitors or statins	Lovastatin (Mevacor) Pravastatin (Pravachol) Simvastatin (Zocor) Fluvastatin (Lescol) Atorvastatin (Lipitor) Rosuvastatin (Crestor)	Mainly lower total cholesterol and LDL cholesterol
Fibrates	Gemfibrozil (Lopid) Fenofibrate (Tricor)	Lower triglycerides. Modest lowering of total cholesterol and LDL cholesterol. Modest increase in HDL cholesterol.
Omega-3 fatty acids	Nutritional supplement	Lower triglycerides. Modest increase in HDL cholesterol.
Niacin (vitamin B_3)	Nutritional supplement	Lowers total cholesterol, LDL cholesterol, and triglycerides. Raises HDL cholesterol.
Ezetimibe	Ezetimibe (Zetia)	Lowers total cholesterol and LDL cholesterol.
Bile acid resins	Cholestyramine (Questran) Colestipol (Cholestid) Colesevelam (Welchol)	Lower total cholesterol and LDL cholesterol; may raise triglycerides.

DID YOU KNOW?

Pancreatitis

There is a genetic defect in some people in whom the triglyceride level can go very high: in the 1,000s (instead of less than 150 mg/dl). This is a serious condition that can lead to an inflammation of the pancreas (**pancreatitis**) and requires hospitalization. The treatment is to stop eating until the triglycerides fall, control the diabetes, and also take one of the fibrate medicines.

DIABETES AND ERECTILE DYSFUNCTION

The ability to get an adequate erection depends upon adequate blood flow to the penis and intact nerve function. Men with diabetes whose nerves to the penis are damaged and/or whose blood supply to the penis is reduced may not be able to get a strong erection. Before blaming nerve damage and blood supply problems for erectile dysfunction, however, it is important to exclude other causes such as low testosterone levels, medicines (for blood pressure and depression), alcohol, and cannabis (marijuana). Psychological issues such as depression, job stress, and other relationship problems may also contribute to erectile dysfunction.

There are a number of treatment options for erectile dysfunction:

- **PDE5 enzyme inhibitors.** Sildenafil (Viagra), vardenafil (Levitra), and tadalafil (Cialis) are the medicines prescribed for erectile dysfunction. These medicines block an enzyme (called cyclic GMP-specific phosphodiesterase type 5), prolonging the blood flow into the penis and so improving the ability to get an erection. When taking these medicines, you do have to be sexually aroused to get an erection. The recommended dose of sildenafil for most patients is one 50-mg tablet taken approximately one hour before sexual activity. The peak effect is at one and a half to two hours, with some effect persisting for four hours. In clinical studies, people with diabetes mellitus using sildenafil reported 50 to 60 percent improvement in erectile function. The recommended doses of both vardenafil and tadalafil are 5 to 20 mg. Tadalafil has been shown to improve erectile function for up to thirty-six hours after dosing. In clinical trials of these medicines, only a few adverse effects were reported—transient mild headache, flushing, dyspepsia, and some altered color vision. If an erection lasts longer than four hours (called **priapism**), you should go to the emergency room. These medicines should not be used if you are taking nitrates for heart disease, because that would cause a severe drop in blood pressure. You should also seek medical advice before taking these medicines if you have heart disease or have had a heart attack, stroke, or a life-threatening heart rhythm problem. Rarely, a decrease in vision or permanent visual loss has been reported after using these drugs.

- **Alprostadil, papaverine, and papaverine with phentolamine.** If the PDE5 inhibitors do not work well, then you can try a medicine called alprostadil, which used to be given by injections, but now is available as a urethral suppository (brand name Muse). It is a tiny pellet that is inserted into the urethra, and it can be quite effective at producing an erection. If this, too, is not successful, then injections into the penis can be tried: the drugs most commonly used include papaverine injection, papaverine with phentolamine injection, and alprostadil (prostaglandin E_1) injection. The injections sound unpleasant but are not that painful. It is important to get careful instructions from your doctor to prevent injury and priapism.

- **External vacuum therapy (Erec-Aid System).** This consists of a suction chamber operated by a hand pump that creates a vacuum around the penis. This draws blood into the penis to produce an erection, which is maintained by a specially designed tension ring inserted around the base of the penis that can be kept in place for up to twenty to thirty minutes. While this method is generally effective, it does require psychological support from the partner.

- If all the treatments described above fail, then surgical implants are available, but rarely needed.

DIABETES AND FEMALE SEXUAL DYSFUNCTION

Women with diabetes are at increased risk for sexual arousal disorder—that is, inadequate vaginal and clitoral swelling in response to sexual arousal. A small research study showed that in women with type 1 diabetes, sildenafil improved arousal, orgasm, and sexual enjoyment. A woman with diabetes should discuss problems of sexual arousal with her physician.

Summary

- The symptoms of diabetes depend upon the degree of insulin deficiency:
  - If the insulin deficiency is modest so that the glucose levels are only slightly elevated, there may be no symptoms and diabetes may be discovered on routine testing.
  - If the insulin deficiency is moderate, the presentation may be of bladder infection, vaginal or penile yeast infection, or increased nighttime urination.
  - If the insulin deficiency is severe, there may be thirst, frequent urination, weight loss, tiredness, and blurred vision. If untreated there can be progression to diabetes ketoacidosis (in type 1 patients) or hyperosmolar coma (in type 2 patients).
- People who have poor glucose control over many years are at risk of developing long-term complications. These include:

- Diabetic eye disease—retinopathy, macular edema, cataracts, glaucoma.
- Untreated diabetic eye disease can lead to blindness.
- Kidney failure, which if severe may lead to dialysis.
- Neuropathy—peripheral neuropathy; autonomic neuropathy with resting fast heart rate and gastroparesis. Diabetic peripheral neuropathy increases the risk of foot injuries and infections. The nerve damage and circulatory problems of the penis can cause erectile dysfunction.
- Circulatory problems: heart disease, strokes, impaired blood flow to the legs.
- Treating blood glucose, lipids, and blood pressure can prevent the development and progression of these complications.

PART TWO

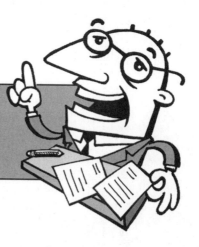

MANAGING YOUR DIABETES DAY-TO-DAY

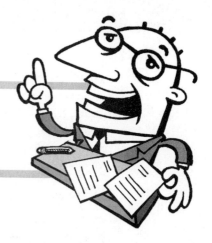

CHAPTER 4

Assembling Your Treatment Team and Support Network

Controlling blood glucose levels successfully takes time and effort. Your illness may affect relationships with your partner, other family members, friends, and colleagues, and you cannot take a holiday from your illness. All of these things can be overwhelming, but with a strong team, you can manage your diabetes. This chapter describes how you can assemble the treatment team and support network that you need for the long-term management of your diabetes.

Educating Yourself

Unlike many other chronic illnesses, diabetes requires significant decision making on a daily basis. I tell my patients that the most important aspect of diabetes care is not what I tell them to do when they see me in my office, but what they do at home. The process of learning how to take care of your diabetes is referred to as **diabetes self-management education (DSME)**.

There are many different ways in which you can obtain the skills and information necessary to take good care of your diabetes, including the following:

- Your medical team
- The American Diabetes Association (ADA)
- WeightWatchers or other weight-loss organizations
- Diabetes support groups
- Books about diabetes
- The Internet

Your Medical Team

Your medical team will provide individual assessment and instruction. Depending on the type of diabetes you have, the resources in your community, and your health plan, your medical team will consist of your primary care physician, a nutritionist, a diabetes educator, a podiatrist, an ophthalmologist, an endocrinologist, and a psychologist or clinical social worker.

PRIMARY CARE PHYSICIAN

Your physician plays a pivotal role in helping you with your diabetes. Usually, she will be the one who makes the diagnosis of diabetes. She will inform you about the kind of diabetes you have and your treatment options. She will screen you for complications and prescribe the medications for diabetes. If you need treatment with insulin, she may also help you adjust the insulin dosage and design the best insulin regimen for you. She will also help coordinate care with the other members of your medical team.

NUTRITIONIST

Having regular consultations with a nutritionist is important for both type 1 and type 2 diabetes patients. The nutritionist will assess your nutritional needs: if you need to lose weight, she will help you to devise a reduced-calorie diet. She will also teach you about foods that raise blood glucose levels and how to count the amount of carbohydrates in your diet. If you have complications of diabetes, she may provide information about foods that are high in fats, cholesterol, protein, potassium, or sodium.

CERTIFIED DIABETES EDUCATOR

The certified diabetes educator (CDE) will educate you about the kind of diabetes you have and your medication options. She will educate you about the importance of controlling glucose, lipids, and blood pressure to prevent complications and about the effects of exercise and emotions on glucose control. She will also show you how to use glucose monitors, how to treat high and low glucose levels, and how to exercise safely. If you are on insulin, she will teach you how to inject insulin and how to use your insulin pens or pumps.

PODIATRIST

If you have evidence for diabetic nerve damage and/or significant circulatory problems, you should visit a **podiatrist** who has an interest and expertise in treating diabetes. If you have diabetic nerve damage or circulation problems, the podiatrist will treat calluses and fungal infections, cut nails, and prescribe orthotic supports or custom shoes as necessary. The podiatrist will also teach you how to look after your feet so that you do not injure them. If you have absolutely normal feet (like many young patients with type 1 diabetes), it is not strictly necessary to see a podiatrist regularly.

OPHTHALMOLOGIST

The **ophthalmologist** will screen you regularly for diabetic eye disease. There is a multitude of evidence to show that with careful follow-up and intervention, vision loss can be avoided in 50 to 90 percent of cases.

ENDOCRINOLOGIST

An **endocrinologist** is a physician who specializes in treatment of the diseases of endocrine glands, including diabetes. In 1999 there were just over four thousand practicing endocrinologists in the United States, and there are about 18 million people with diabetes, so only a very small number of people with diabetes will ever see an endocrinologist. You should think about having an endocrinologist review your diabetes care if

- Despite your and your medical team's best efforts you are not able to get your glucose levels under target.
- You need help treating low-glucose reactions or you have had hospital admissions for your diabetes.
- You have type 1 diabetes or an unusual form of diabetes.

PSYCHOLOGIST, PSYCHIATRIST, OR CLINICAL SOCIAL WORKER

Fitting diabetes care into the whole scheme of a busy life can be quite difficult, and it is often helpful if you have someone to talk to. Studies have shown that depression is twice as common in people with diabetes, and a psychologist or psychiatrist can evaluate and treat you for depression if necessary. Your clinical social worker can provide individual therapy.

OTHER MEDICAL PROVIDERS

If you have other complications of diabetes, you may see other providers such as a cardiologist, a nephrologist, a dermatologist, a rheumatologist, or a hand surgeon. Your primary care physician can make the appropriate referrals to these medical specialists.

Choosing Your Medical Team

How can you find out whether your health-care provider and medical team are giving you the very best care for your diabetes? This is a difficult question to answer. In assessing your physician's ability to manage your diabetes adequately, consider the following:

- **Is your physician interested?** Does your physician talk to you about your diabetes and related issues? Is she interested in hearing about your concerns about the disease, and does she include you in the decision-making process? Your physician should spend time with you to create a treatment plan for your diabetes.
- **Does your physician follow the American Diabetes Association guidelines?** You can find these guidelines through the ADA website (diabetes.org) or the website for the ADA's journal *Diabetes Care* (http://

care.diabetesjournals.org/content/vaol30/suppl_1). Does your doctor talk to you about them and do tests and evaluations at the recommended intervals?

- **Does your physician encourage you to become an expert in your own diabetes?** Has she referred you to see a nutritionist, visit a diabetes educator, and attend diabetes self-help classes at your local hospital?

- **Is your physician willing to give recommendations for you to see other specialists?** If you think that you need to see a heart specialist or endocrinologist, is she willing to make a referral?

- **Are you and your physician compatible?** Do you feel that you have a good relationship with your doctor? Does she respect you, and do you respect her?

You can ask similar questions about the other providers as well. Word of mouth from other people with diabetes in your community is helpful in finding the good doctors and other medical programs. There may also be ADA-certified programs in your area. As with everything else, the more you know about a subject, the easier it is for you to assess the quality and expertise of someone else on that subject.

The ADA and Other Sources of Diabetes-Related Information

The American Diabetes Association has an excellent website, and it also publishes many self-help books for patients. You can also seek out local diabetes support groups through your local hospital or pharmacist or by searching on the Internet. There are support groups that cater to people with type 1 and type 2 diabetes, those using insulin pumps, and families who have children with diabetes. These groups enable people with diabetes to share experiences and enhance their knowledge about diabetes self-management.

There are also many Internet websites devoted to diabetes. They vary in the quality of information they provide, so you may want to go to the websites of professional organizations like the ADA first. You can also look at the Canadian Diabetes Association and the British Diabetes Association websites (see Resources). Once you get good basic information, then you can go to websites that cater to specific issues like insulin pumps or diabetes and exercise. Information about diabetes medications changes rapidly, and there is usually good information at the website of the manufacturer of a particular drug.

Setting Up a Support Network

When you are diagnosed with a chronic illness like diabetes, you may go through a period of grief because of the loss of good health. The diagnosis can be overwhelming: there is a lot of information that you need to grasp—you have to learn about carbohydrates, calories, exercise, weight management, and checking blood glucose levels. You may need to take oral medications or inject insulin. You may also have some or all of these questions:

- What impact will this have on my family?
- How will it affect my job?
- How will it affect my sex life?
- How and what do I tell my family, friends, and colleagues?
- Do I have to check my blood glucose levels in public?
- Can I drive?
- Will I go blind?
- Does this mean that I will have to go on dialysis?
- Will I lose my leg?
- Am I going to die?

You may feel anxious, or you might panic or go emotionally numb. You might decide to ignore the whole thing and hope the diabetes will go away. Or you might get angry—why me? You might blame the doctor for not picking up the problem sooner. You may feel that your partner or family members will not understand. Eventually you may come to terms with your diabetes: you don't have to like having it, but you decide that within the limitations placed by the diabetes, you are going to make the best of it.

These emotions of shock, denial, anger, and acceptance upon being diagnosed with diabetes may happen at different times and with different intensity. Even after accepting that you have diabetes, there is the continued stress of looking after this chronic condition, and depression is more common in people with diabetes.

Clinical research shows that people who have a strong support network go through these phases of grief better than those who try to do it alone. The support can be emotional (for example, someone to lean on when you are discouraged) or practical (for example, help treating low glucose levels, assistance with meal plans, or an exercise partner who provides encouragement to stick with an exercise plan).

There is no one way to setting up such a support network, but here are some suggestions:

- Identify a close family member or friend with whom you can share your thoughts and emotions.

- Get your family members well informed about your kind of diabetes and involve them in your care. Explain the benefits of your diet and exercise plan and have family members follow these plans, too.

- Start talking and making connections with other people with diabetes.

- Express to your friends and family how much you appreciate their support.

- Be proactive about your health care:

  - Seek out medical care providers who will give you the right advice.

  - Join patient advocacy groups like the ADA and the JDF (Juvenile Diabetes Foundation) (see Resources).

Summary

- With careful planning, a positive attitude, and support from your medical team and your friends and family, you can manage your diabetes and live well. Your medical support team includes:

  - Your physician, who will diagnose and monitor your diabetes, prescribe medicines, and refer you to other specialists as necessary.

  - The nutritionist, who will explain how food affects your glucose levels, teach carbohydrate counting, and help with weight-loss strategies.

  - The diabetes educator, who will teach you how to inject insulin, monitor blood glucose, and treat low glucose reactions.

  - The podiatrist, who will screen you for diabetic nerve damage and teach you how to avoid foot injury.

  - The ophthalmologist, who will screen you for diabetic eye disease.

  - The endocrinologist, if you have type 1 diabetes or an unusual form of diabetes, or if you are having lots of problems controlling your diabetes.

  - The psychologist or clinical social worker, if you're having trouble adjusting emotionally to the demands of your disease.

- Your social support team includes:

  - Family and friends who can provide emotional support and help you with your care.

  - The wider diabetes community—other people with diabetes in your neighborhood, the Internet community, and advocacy groups like the ADA and JDF.

CHAPTER 5

Monitoring Your Diabetes

The goals of diabetes management are to control blood glucose levels and to screen and treat related conditions such as high blood pressure, lipid abnormalities, high cholesterol, and other complications of diabetes. This means that you will need to learn how to monitor your blood glucose levels, and you will also have more frequent laboratory tests and visits to your doctor than do people without diabetes. This chapter tells you both how you will monitor your glucose levels and what other tests your doctor may do to evaluate your diabetes.

Monitoring Glucose Levels

When you have diabetes, your glucose levels fluctuate much more than those of people without diabetes. In people without diabetes, fasting glucose levels in the morning are usually between 60 and 100 mg/dl. Before each meal, the levels are below 100 mg/dl. The peak values one to two hours after a meal are in the 120s and usually stay below 140, even after a meal rich in carbohydrates.

With current therapies, it is difficult to achieve normal glucose levels when you have diabetes. Even when levels are below 100 mg/dl before meals, they frequently go above the 140 range after meals. This is especially true if you take insulin, in which case aiming for normal glucose levels can significantly increase the risk of hypoglycemia (see Chapter 7). The only time doctors attempt to achieve normal glucose levels in insulin-treated patients is during pregnancy, when the target for premeal blood glucose level is 60 to 100 mg/dl, postmeal peak level (usually about one and a half to two hours after a meal) is less than 130 mg/dl, and bedtime and 2 A.M. levels are around 100 mg/dl.

If you are insulin-treated and are not pregnant, your doctor will aim for premeal glucose levels between 90 and 130 mg/dl and postmeal levels less than 180 mg/dl.

These targets are just general guidelines and will vary from person to person. Some people can and do achieve much lower levels, whereas for others these targets are too tight, and they will get unacceptably frequent low glucose reactions.

Table 5-1 sums up the ADA's recommendations for blood glucose targets.

UNDERSTANDING HOME MONITORING

Blood glucose monitoring at home is an important part of diabetes management and serves a number of purposes. First, monitoring at home makes it easier to detect low blood glucose reactions, because you cannot rely on how you feel to detect low glucose levels. When aiming for the glucose targets mentioned in Table 5-1, many people with diabetes develop hypoglycemic unawareness (see Chapter 7), meaning they can have glucose levels in the 40s and 50s and still feel quite fine. For this reason,

Table 5-1 Blood-Glucose Target Levels			
	Normal Levels (mg/dl)	**Targets During Pregnancy Complicated by Diabetes (mg/dl)**	**Targets for Patients Who Are Not Pregnant (mg/dl)**
Fasting and premeal	Less than 100 (often 70s or low 80s)	60 to 100	90 to 130
Postmeal	Less than 140 (often 120s)	Less than 130	Less than 180
Bedtime	Less than 100 (often 70s or low 80s)	100	100 to 130

measuring glucose levels frequently allows detection and treatment before the glucose levels fall too low. This monitoring is particularly relevant when exercising or when performing activities such as driving or operating machinery, when you need to be alert.

Second, home monitoring allows you to detect high glucose levels. Elevated glucose levels may reflect dietary indiscretion or failure to take or to adjust diabetes medications. If you are on an insulin pump, there is not a big depot of insulin in the subcutaneous tissues, and if for any reason the insulin delivery gets interrupted, glucose levels can go very high and DKA (see Chapter 3) can develop over a few hours. Persistently elevated high glucose levels increase the risk of developing long-term complications of diabetes.

Finally, home monitoring allows you to adjust medication doses, particularly insulin. If you're an insulin-treated patient, check your blood glucose levels at least four times or more a day. If you have type 2 diabetes controlled with diet only or are on medications that do not cause low glucose levels (for example, metformin, pioglitazone, rosiglitazone, or exenatide), checking blood glucose levels a few times a week may suffice. However, if you have type 2 diabetes and are taking oral medicines that can cause low glucose levels (sulfonylureas, repaglinide, and nateglinide), one or two blood glucose checks per day are necessary.

USING A HOME GLUCOSE METER

At least twenty-eight different home blood glucose meters are available in the United States. All are accurate, but they vary in their features:

- Size of display screen and backlight, which is important if you have visual problems
- Step-by-step voice guide and ability to give verbal results, which is important if you're visually impaired
- Size of blood drop required
- The ease with which blood can be placed on the glucose test strip that measures the glucose level
- The ability of the system to sense whether the blood sample is insufficient
- The need to calibrate each batch of glucose strips being used by entering a code
- Speed with which you get the results, ranging from five to thirty seconds
- The number of glucose values that can be stored in the memory
- The ability of the meter to display glucose results graphically

- Software to download the data to your computer
- The ability to flag results with comments about carbohydrates, insulin doses, or exercise
- How much cleaning and maintenance is needed

Glucose meters are relatively inexpensive, ranging from fifty to one hundred dollars each. Test strips are the major expense, however, costing fifty to seventy-five cents each. Most health insurance covers the costs of the strips, but the actual amount of coverage will depend on your plan. Medicare, for example, covers strips for one check a day if you are not on insulin and four checks a day if you are on insulin. Your doctor can help you get more strips if necessary.

Here are some additional monitoring tips:

- **Cleaning your hands:** Before testing, wash your hands, because lotions and other residues can affect the results. You do not, however, need to clean your fingertips with alcohol.

- **Coding your meter:** Your meter may require you to enter a code for each new batch of strips (the number is on the container), or it may need you to insert a code chip that comes with each batch of strips. Failure to follow the proper coding procedure for your meter will give you inaccurate results. Meters are also supplied with control solutions—the outside of your glucose strip container has the range of numbers that you should get when

DID YOU KNOW?

How Glucose Meters Work

A glucose meter is a battery-operated handheld device the size of a pager with a display screen and a hole to insert a thin plastic glucose test strip, which measures about one inch by one-quarter inch. Most meters turn on when you insert the test strip. You prick your finger, you touch the blood drop with the tip or side of the test strip, and the blood is drawn up into the strip by capillary action. The chemicals that are in the strip then react with the glucose in the blood and produce a tiny electrical current. The meter measures the electrical current, which is proportional to the glucose concentration in the blood sample, and the data is displayed on the screen as a glucose number. The test strip is then discarded, and a new one is used each time you check your blood glucose level.

you measure the glucose in the control solution. You need to use the control solution from time to time to make sure that the meter is giving accurate readings. If you run out of the control solution, call the manufacturer for more.

- **Obtaining blood:** Each glucose meter comes with a **lancet** device and disposable 26- to 33-gauge lancets. Many lancet devices allow you to adjust the puncture depth so that you can make sure you can get an adequate blood drop. You can reuse the lancets, but you must not share the same lancet with friends or family because of the risk of transmitting a blood-borne viral illness. Remember, pricking your fingers on the side hurts less than if you prick the tip of your finger.

- **Choosing an alternate testing site:** Quite a few meters have been approved for checking blood glucose in the forearm or thigh. However, you may want to avoid testing at these alternate sites because there is a five- to twenty-minute lag in the glucose response on the arm compared to the fingertip. If you are checking to find out whether you are hypoglycemic, you definitely want to know what the number is *now*, not what it was five to twenty minutes ago.

- **Avoiding expired test strips:** Do not use expired testing strips, and always close the strip containers properly after each use. Out-of-date strips and improperly stored strips may give inaccurate results.

- **Obtaining accurate readings across the glucose range:** All meters and the test strips are calibrated for glucose concentrations ranging from 60 to 160 mg/dl, but accuracy is not as good for glucose levels higher and lower than this range. When blood glucose is less than 60 mg/dl, the difference between the meter and the laboratory value may be as much as 20 percent. Keep this in mind if your levels fall above or below 60 to 160 mg/dl.

- **Identifying whole blood versus plasma glucose levels:** Be aware that some older meters (such as the One Touch Profile) are calibrated against whole blood glucose concentrations, which means that displayed values are 10 to 15 percent lower than the laboratory glucose result. This is not true for many new meters, which are calibrated against plasma glucose.

- **Converting the metric system:** In Europe and some other parts of the world, glucose is measured in SI units (millimoles per liter, written as mmol/L) rather than in milligrams per deciliter (mg/dl) as is done in the United States. To convert from mg/dl to mmol/L, divide by 18. For example, a glucose measurement of 100 mg/dl is the same as 5.5 mmol/L (100/18 = 5.5). If you buy a glucose meter in Europe, the results will be displayed in mmol/L. Do not confuse a reading of 5.5 on a European meter as 55 mg/dl! Some meters can be switched to show glucose levels in mg/dl or mmol/L, and it is important that you do not inadvertently switch the readings from mg/dl to mmol/L and misinterpret the glucose levels. Most new meters that are now being sold in the United States no longer allow this conversion.

• **Monitoring if you are anemic or are on supplemental oxygen:** Suffering from severe anemia or being on supplemental oxygen can affect the readings on some glucose meters. So if you suffer from severe anemia or are on supplemental oxygen, check with the manufacturer of your meter to see whether your results will be affected.

• **Solving problems with your meter:** If your meter is not working well or you are having problems, call the toll-free telephone number provided on the back of the meter, and the representatives at the meter company will help you.

RECORDING YOUR BLOOD GLUCOSE

To keep track of your blood glucose (BG) values, you have two options: you can write down the numbers in a blood glucose diary, or you can download the data from your meter into your computer and take them to the doctor's office for analysis. Even if you cannot write down numbers regularly, do so for a week before you go to see your doctor. Figure 5-1 is an example of a blood glucose log for someone who monitors glucose levels a few times a day.

Downloading the data to your computer may seem like less work, but there are a few disadvantages to this approach:

Figure 5-1 Blood Glucose Log

Time	12 A.M.					6 A.M.					12 P.M.					6 P.M.
BG																
CHO																
Insulin for CHO																
Insulin for high BG																
Basal insulin																
Comments																

- First and most important, your tendency may be to download data into the computer and print it out just before your doctor's visit. This is not as helpful because you do not review data as it is generated, and so you do not intervene between office visits. On the other hand, if you write down the numbers, it is very easy for you review the data as you go along, looking for patterns and making interventions as necessary.

- Second, if you do not enter insulin dosage, carbohydrate intake, and other factors such as exercise that might have affected a particular glucose level, it is difficult to put the downloaded glucose values in context.

- Third, meter manufacturers each have their own software, and quite often the software does not display data in formats that are easy to analyze.

Even if you keep a pen-and-paper log, your doctor may periodically review the BG numbers in your meter's memory if he or she believes you aren't recording accurately. Sometimes people don't write down very high or low glucose values, in an attempt to make their diabetes appear better than it is.

USING CONTINUOUS GLUCOSE MONITORING SYSTEMS

With conventional home blood glucose monitors, depending on how many times you prick your finger, you may check your glucose levels anywhere from one to twelve times per day. New kinds of monitoring systems, called continuous glucose monitoring systems, are now available that measure glucose levels every few minutes throughout the day and night. These systems enable you to review your glucose levels overnight while you are asleep and also trend glucose changes following food, insulin injections, and exercise. The three systems currently on the market are made

DID YOU KNOW?

Measuring Glucose in the Urine

It is possible to measure glucose in the urine with urine testing strips called Diastix or Clinistix. However, because glucose appears in the urine only if the blood glucose levels are over 200, this approach cannot allow you to achieve the recommended glucose targets given in Table 5-1. Therefore, urine glucose measurements are no longer recommended for treatment of diabetes.

by DexCom, MiniMed Medtronic, and Animas. An additional one made by Abbott Pharmaceuticals (called the Navigator) is being reviewed by the FDA and should become available in the near future, as will other models after the publication of this book. Check with your doctor for up-to-date information on the latest systems.

The DexCom, Medtronic, and Abbott Systems

The DexCom, Medtronic MiniMed, and Abbott Pharmaceutical (not yet available) systems all work in a similar way. The sensor is a tiny flexible probe that you insert under the skin in the same way you insert an insulin pump infusion set cannula (see Chapter 6). The sensor measures the glucose concentration in the tissue fluid every five minutes for about three to seven days before it needs replacing. All the systems have software available to download the data into your computer.

These systems are not covered by insurance, and the initial cost for the two systems that are currently available is about $800 to $1,000. The main expense, however, is the sensor, which has to be changed every three to seven days. The three-day sensor costs about $35. This adds up to an out-of-pocket expense of about $4,000 annually.

These systems enable some patients to improve control without increasing the risk of hypoglycemia. The individual blood glucose values are not that critical; what matters is that the system alerts you to the direction and the rate at which the glucose level is changing, allowing you to take corrective action. You learn how different foods get absorbed and how quickly your glucose rises after a meal. You can use this information to change the timing and the ratio of insulin for carbohydrates to control the glucose rise. The other main benefit is in alerting you to low glucose levels. Spouses and friends report that they especially appreciate the low glucose alerts.

With the DexCom system, the measured glucose values are transmitted to a separate pager-like device with a screen, with alerts for low and high values. The screen of the DexCom device graphically displays the glucose levels for the previous nine hours. It also displays the last glucose number.

With the MiniMed system, you have the option of having the data wirelessly transmitted to the screen of an insulin pump, again with alerts for high and low values. This system graphically displays the glucose levels for the previous twenty-four hours and the last glucose value. Unlike the DexCom system, the MiniMed system also allows you to scroll back to see actual numbers for previous glucose levels rather than just a graphic display.

Both the DexCom and MiniMed systems require you to calibrate the machines with periodic finger-prick glucose levels. There are concerns regarding reliability of the values, and so you do need to check your blood glucose with your home blood glucose monitor before making interventions such as injecting extra insulin or eating extra carbohydrates.

The GlucoWatch System

The GlucoWatch system from Animas Technologies measures glucose in the tissue fluid extracted through intact skin by applying a low electric current (a process called reverse iontophoresis). This process can cause local skin irritation, and sweating can cause frequent skipped results. For these reasons, the system is not popular.

Additional Tests to Evaluate Your Diabetes

In addition to monitoring glucose, other tests help you monitor your diabetes.

MONITORING HBA1C

The **hemoglobin H1c (HbA1c)** test (also called the **A1c** test and **glycohemoglobin** test) estimates your glucose control over the previous three to four months and is used by your doctor to assess your overall glucose control. The HbA1c test measures the amount of glucose that is attached to the hemoglobin (the oxygen-carrying protein) in the red blood cells. You can think of HbA1c as "sugar coating" on the hemoglobin—the higher the average glucose levels in your bloodstream, the higher the thickness of the sugar coating; that is, the more glucose is attached to the hemoglobin. Once the glucose is attached to the hemoglobin it stays there for the lifetime of the red cell, which is 120 days. Thus, measuring the amount of glucose attached to the hemoglobin in the blood gives you an estimate of the average glucose levels in the previous three to four months.

An average glucose increase of 35 mg/dl raises the HbA1c by 1 percent. Thus, if your average glucose levels are around 200, you will have an HbA1c of around 8. It has been shown that an elevated HbA1c is associated with increased risk for development of long-term diabetes complications. The ADA recommends that most people with diabetes have an HbA1c between 6 and 7. The reason for this cutoff is that with HbA1c levels in this range, you have a relatively low risk for severe long-term complications, whereas aiming for lower values would significantly increase the risk of hypoglycemic reactions.

Table 5-2 illustrates the relationship between HbA1c levels and average glucose levels.

HbA1c (%)	Mean Plasma Glucose Level (mg/dl)
4	65
5	100
6	135
7	170
8	205
9	240
10	275
11	310
12	345

Table 5-2   HbA1c Levels and Average Glucose Levels

Source: Rohlfing CL, Wiedmeyer HM, Little RR, England JD, Tennill A, Goldstein DE. "Defining the relationship between plasma glucose and HbA(1c): analysis of glucose profiles and HbA(1c) in the Diabetes Control and Complications Trial." *Diabetes Care* 2002; 25: 275–78.

Your doctor will measure the HbA1c level at least three to four times a year. If the value is above the recommended range, he or she will work with you to lower glucose levels further by making additional changes to your diet, exercise program, and diabetes medications.

HbA1c values will be artificially low if you have medical conditions that decrease the life of the red blood cells. Blood transfusions, gastrointestinal bleeding, and some blood cell conditions such as beta thalassemia major are examples of medical conditions in which the HbA1c levels do not reflect the blood glucose levels.

If the HbA1c value is not likely to be accurate, your doctor may instead do another test called **fructosamine** level. This measures the glucose attachment on other proteins in the blood (plasma proteins), the principal one being albumin. Your doctor will use the fructosamine level in the same way as the HbA1c test result: to guide therapy.

MEASURING KETONES

Ketones are chemicals made by the liver when the body uses fat for energy. If your diabetes goes severely out of control, ketone levels can rise excessively in the blood and urine. This can occur with illnesses such as a bad case of the flu or a gastrointestinal infection or pneumonia. It can also occur when people with type 1 diabetes forget to take their insulin, if the insulin goes bad, or if their insulin pump malfunctions. High ketone levels with nausea or vomiting indicates possible DKA, and medical evaluation and hospital treatment may be necessary.

You can measure ketones in the urine using ketone strips (Acetest, Ketostix), or you can measure it on a blood drop just like glucose using the Precision Xtra glucose meter (made by Abbott), which not only measures glucose but also measures one of the blood ketones called beta-hydroxybutyrate using special strips. Since beta-hydroxybutyrate is the major ketone in DKA, this is the preferred test. Beta-hydroxybutyrate levels below 0.6 mmol/L are considered normal, and levels above 1.5 mmol/L are of concern for DKA.

If you have type 1 diabetes, you should measure your ketones if your blood glucose levels are unexpectedly high (more than 250 mg/dl) and won't come down and/or you feel ill with nausea, vomiting, or dizziness. Table 5-3 summarizes what you should do in these cases.

MONITORING BLOOD PRESSURE

Blood pressure control is critical for the prevention of both microvascular and macrovascular complications of diabetes. The goal should be to have blood pressure measurements consistently below 130/80. Sometimes you may find that the blood pressure is high only when you see a doctor or when you see a particular doctor (a phenomenon called white-coat hypertension). If this is the case, ask to have your blood pressure measured when you see other doctors, or buy a home blood pressure machine and use those blood pressure measurements as a guide to treatment. Blood pressure is often easier to control than blood glucose levels, and controlling blood pressure is just as beneficial to your health. You doctor may not routinely recommend measuring blood pressure at home unless there is a suggestion that you have white-coat hypertension or symptoms that might be due to low or high blood pressure.

Table 5-3 Guidelines for Treatment of Ketones in Type 1 Diabetes	
If BG persistently over 250 mg/dl and blood ketones less than 1.5 or urine ketones absent or small	**If BG persistently over 250 mg/dl and blood ketones above 1.5 or urine ketones moderate to large**
Drink plenty of fluids. Give fast-acting insulin. Monitor glucose levels.	Call medical team for advice or go to the emergency room. Drink plenty of fluids. Give fast-acting insulin. Monitor glucose and ketone levels.

MONITORING LIPIDS (CHOLESTEROL LEVELS)

Heart disease is a risk factor in people with diabetes, especially if you have type 2 diabetes, long-standing type 1 diabetes, or complications from type 1 diabetes. In type 2 diabetes, the risk of heart attack is increased twofold. This is the same frequency as nondiabetic individuals who have already had a previous heart attack. Under these circumstances, your LDL cholesterol should be below 100 mg/dl—ideally around 70 mg/dl. Have your lipid levels checked annually by your physician, and more frequently if you are getting treated. If you are a young patient with type 1 diabetes and your lipid profile is normal, measuring your lipids every two years is fine.

MONITORING KIDNEY FUNCTION

Screening for kidney disease is very important because there are treatments that prevent the kidney disease from getting worse (see Chapter 3). The screening usually starts five years after diagnosis in people with type 1 diabetes, and at diagnosis in people with type 2 diabetes. The ADA recommends that people with diabetes be screened annually for kidney disease by measuring blood creatinine levels and urine albumin level in the first morning urine. It is not necessary to do a twenty-four-hour or an overnight urine collection: the spot urine first thing in the morning is just as good. Your doctor will give you a small urine cup, and you will collect the first morning urine and take it to the lab. A urine albumin of less than 30 (milligrams per gram creatinine) is normal, 30 to 300 indicates early diabetic kidney disease (microalbuminuria), and greater than 300 indicates more significant disease (macroalbuminuria).

The urine albumin test is affected by posture and physical activity, and it is important to collect the first morning urine immediately after you get up. Fever and uncontrolled diabetes with very high glucose levels can also falsely raise the urine albumin excretion, and so you should wait until these problems have resolved before doing the test. If there is a marginal elevation in the urine albumin excretion, your doctor will measure it again within the next six months.

MONITORING FOR DIABETIC EYE DISEASE

The ADA recommends that people with diabetes get regular eye examinations. The screening starts five years after diagnosis in people with type 1 diabetes and at diagnosis in people with type 2 diabetes. The frequency of the eye examinations depends a little bit on the age of the patient, duration of diabetes, and the presence of complications. At a minimum, have a comprehensive eye examination by an ophthalmologist or optometrist every two years.

MONITORING FOR DIABETIC FOOT DISEASE

Your doctor should examine your feet once a year to check for injuries due to diabetes. If you're at higher risk for foot injury—that is, if you have severe nerve damage (and can't feel pieces of grit in your shoe), calluses, altered foot shape, a previous foot ulcer, or circulatory problems—regularly see a podiatrist for evaluation, treatment, and education.

SCREENING FOR THYROID DISEASE

People with type 1 diabetes are at higher risk for autoimmune thyroid disease—most frequently the thyroid is underactive (Hashimoto's thyroiditis), but it can also sometimes be overactive (Graves' disease). Your doctor will check you for thyroid disease when you are first diagnosed with type 1 diabetes and then every one to two years. Thyroid abnormalities also increase with age, and your doctor therefore may do thyroid tests periodically even if you have type 2 diabetes.

Summary

- Home blood glucose monitoring allows you to
  - Assess your glucose levels in response to food, exercise, and medications
  - Adjust your insulin and avoid dangerously low glucose reactions
- Continuous glucose monitoring systems measure glucose levels every five minutes around the clock, and you can see the trends in your glucose levels in response to food, exercise, and medications.
- Your HbA1c level is an assessment of overall glucose control, and your doctor will measure it every three to four months.
- To keep the complications of diabetes at bay, your doctor will
  - Monitor your blood pressure
  - Monitor your lipid levels
  - Monitor your kidney function
  - Screen you for neuropathy
  - Check you for thyroid problems
- An ophthalmologist or optometrist should monitor you for diabetic eye disease each year.

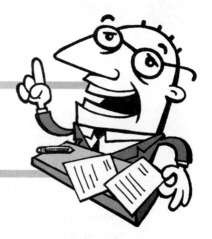

CHAPTER 6

Medicine for Diabetes

To treat your diabetes successfully, you will need to have some familiarity with the medicines that are currently available. In this chapter, I talk specifically about the medications that control blood glucose levels. Medicines to treat complications of diabetes, such as high blood pressure and high lipid levels, are discussed in Chapter 3.

Diabetes Medications 101

Let me make a few general comments about diabetes medications before I discuss them in detail in the following sections.

Medicines for diabetes are only one component of the treatment of diabetes. To be successful in controlling the diabetes, you also need to consider other aspects of diabetes care, such as diet and exercise. Whether a specific medicine is suitable for you depends on:

- The type of diabetes you have
- The other medical problems you may have, which can prevent the use of certain medicines
- The side effects you may experience with a particular medicine

Your doctor may have differing experiences with the medicine, and this may influence which ones he or she prescribes.

The discussion of medicines is complicated by the fact that each drug has at least two names—the proprietary or brand name given by the pharmaceutical company and the generic name. After the pharmaceutical company patent runs out, a number of less expensive generic versions of the medicine become available. In my experience, generic diabetes medicines work just fine, and if one is available, I would switch to a generic drug. The tables in this chapter list the medicines by the generic names and the brand names. In the text of this chapter and the rest of the book, I refer to the medicines by the generic names rather than the brand names.

If a medicine has the letters XR, ER, LA, CR, or SR, it means that the drug is in a slow-release form.

- XR and ER refer to extended release
- LA refers to long acting
- CR refers to controlled release
- SR refers to slow release

In people with type 1 diabetes and some other types of diabetes where the principal problem is beta cell failure and decreased insulin secretion, the treatment is to replace the insulin. There are many types of insulin, and I describe them in the "Insulin" section later in this chapter.

Type 2 diabetes is different in that there are multiple factors that contribute to the elevated glucose levels (see Chapter 2). These factors include:

- Inadequate insulin secretion
- Increased production of glucose by the liver
- Resistance of the tissues to insulin action
- Obesity and excess caloric intake

The medicines for type 2 diabetes target these various factors, and I first talk about them.

Medicines for Type 2 Diabetes

Common medications for diabetes are discussed in the following sections.

SULFONYLUREAS, REPAGLINIDE, AND NATEGLINIDE

How They Work

These are oral medications (see Table 6-1) that bind to receptors on the beta cell, causing it to release insulin. The released insulin then lowers the glucose levels.

Tolbutamide, chlorpropamide, acetohexamide, and tolazamide are referred to as first-generation sulfonylureas, and, with the exception of tolbutamide, are rarely used these days. The newer, second-generation drugs are glyburide, glipizide, glimepiride, and gliclazide, and these are commonly used. They vary in their duration of effect and how they are removed from the body.

Nateglinide and repaglinide are chemically different from the sulfonylureas, but they work the same way. Their effect lasts only a few hours, and so they are commonly given before each meal.

Side Effects

The main side effect of these medicines is that they can cause hypoglycemia (low blood glucose reactions) if a person takes the prescribed dose and does not eat enough. The risk of hypoglycemia with the sulfonylureas is higher in the elderly and those with kidney failure. For these groups, it is better to use lower doses and the fast-acting drugs—glipizide, repaglinide, and nateglinide. Tolbutamide is also an inexpensive option that can be given two or three times a day and has a low risk of hypoglycemia.

People taking these medicines tend to gain some weight with time. The reasons for the weight gain are not clear—one possibility is that at times the medicine causes low glucose levels, causing hunger so that the person overeats. Also, perhaps if the person sees that the medicine controls the glucose level well, he or she might be tempted to eat more, thinking that there will not be any consequences.

Generic Drug Name (Brand Name in Parentheses)	**Strength**	**Daily Dose**
Table 6-1 Oral Diabetes Medicines That Stimulate Insulin Release		
Sulfonylureas		
Tolbutamide (Orinase)	500 mg	0.5–2 g in 2 or 3 divided doses
Tolazamide (Tolinase)	100, 250, and 500 mg	0.1–1 g as single dose or in 2 divided doses
Acetohexamide (Dymelor)	250 and 500 mg	0.25–1.5 g as single dose or in 2 divided doses
Chlorpropamide (Diabinese)	100 and 250 mg	0.1–0.5 g as single dose
Glyburide (Diabeta, Micronase)	1.25, 2.5, and 5 mg	1.25–20 mg as single dose or in 2 divided doses
Slow-release glyburide (Glynase)	1.5, 3, and 6 mg	1.5–18 mg as single dose or in 2 divided doses
Glipizide (Glucotrol)	5 and 10 mg	2.5–40 mg as single dose or in 2 divided doses on an empty stomach
Slow-release glipizide (Glucotrol XL)	5 and 10 mg	Up to 20 or 30 mg daily as a single dose
Gliclazide	80 mg	40–80 mg as single dose; 160–320 mg as divided dose (not available in U.S.)
Glimepiride (Amaryl)	1, 2, and 4 mg	1–4 mg as single dose; 8 mg as divided dose
D-phenylalanine derivative		
Nateglinide (Starlix)	60 and 120 mg	60 to 120 mg 3 times a day; lasts for up to 1.5 hours
Meglitinide analog		
Repaglinide (Prandin)	0.5, 1, and 2 mg	4 mg in up to 3 divided doses given 15 minutes before a meal; lasts for up to 3 hours

METFORMIN

How It Works

The liver of a person with type 2 diabetes releases too much glucose into the blood-stream. Metformin (see Table 6-2) works to reduce the glucose production by the liver.

Table 6-2	Oral Diabetes Medicines That Decrease Glucose Release from the Liver	
Generic Drug Name (Brand Name in Parentheses)	**Strength**	**Daily Dose**
Biguanides		
Metformin (Glucophage)	500, 850, and 1,000 mg	Maximum 850 mg three times a day; most doctors use 1,000 mg twice a day as a maximal dose
Extended-release metformin (Glucophage XR)	500 and 750 mg	Maximum 2,000 mg once a day

Unlike the sulfonylureas, metformin does not stimulate insulin release from the beta cells, and so it does not cause hypoglycemia. In fact, in people taking metformin alone, the glucose levels and the insulin levels are both lower. Metformin also reduces appetite and promotes weight loss, and it has a beneficial effect on some risk factors for heart disease such as lowering triglycerides. In a large clinical study of people with type 2 diabetes (called the United Kingdom Prospective Diabetes Study or UKPDS), metformin treatment in obese individuals was found to be more effective than insulin or sulfonylureas in reducing heart attacks. Therefore, metformin is the first-line therapy for type 2 diabetes.

Side Effects

The main side effects of metformin are nausea and occasionally diarrhea. You can limit these side effects by taking the medicine with food and starting at a low dose. The side effects are also dose dependent, and some people can tolerate only a low dose.

Rarely, people taking metformin can develop a serious medical condition called **lactic acidosis**, which can lead to death and so requires immediate hospitalization. The symptoms of lactic acidosis include nausea, vomiting, abdominal pain, rapid breathing, and feeling very unwell. People with liver failure, kidney failure, or severe heart failure are at a higher risk for lactic acidosis and therefore should not take this medicine.

Table 6-3 Oral Diabetes Medicines That Block the Activity of Enzymes That Break Down Starches		
Generic Drug Name (Brand Name in Parentheses)	**Strength**	**Daily Dose**
Alpha-glucosidase inhibitors		
Acarbose (Precose)	50 and 100 mg	75 to 300 mg in 3 divided doses before each meal; lasts 4 hours
Miglitol (Glyset)	25, 50, and 100 mg	75 to 300 mg in 3 divided doses before each meal; lasts 4 hours

ACARBOSE AND MIGLITOL (ALPHA-GLUCOSIDASE INHIBITORS)

How They Work

These medications (see Table 6-3) partially block the enzymes in the small-bowel wall that break down starches, so that the glucose rise after eating starchy foods is delayed and the glucose peak is lower.

Side Effects

When you take these medicines, more starch breakdown products find their way to the lower part of the bowel and the action of the intestinal bacteria on these starches leads to production of gas (flatulence) and abdominal discomfort. The effects of these medicines on overall glucose levels are modest, and with the availability of other, more effective medicine for diabetes, their use is somewhat limited. Miglitol should not be used in people with kidney failure.

ROSIGLITAZONE AND PIOGLITAZONE

These medications are also called thiazolidinediones, TZDs, or glitazones.

How They Work

These are insulin sensitizers: they work by making the tissues more sensitive to the effects of insulin (see Table 6-4).

Table 6-4	Oral Diabetes Medicines That Work by Making Tissues More Sensitive to Insulin	
Generic Drug Name (Brand Name in Parentheses)	**Strength**	**Daily Dose**
Thiazolidinediones		
Rosiglitazone (Avandia)	2, 4, and 8 mg	2 to 8 mg once a day (or in 2 divided doses)
Pioglitazone (ACTOS)	15, 30, and 45 mg	15 to 45 mg once a day

They usually take a few days to work, so you should not expect glucose levels to fall for at least a week or two. The medicine does depend on having enough insulin to be effective. In addition to their glucose-lowering effect, thiazolidinediones lower triglycerides and free fatty acid levels and raise total cholesterol, LDL cholesterol, and HDL cholesterol. Pioglitazone, when compared to rosiglitazone, is more effective in lowering triglycerides and raising HDL cholesterol. It also does not raise LDL cholesterol as much as rosiglitazone does. Since lipid abnormalities are associated with heart disease, it has been proposed that the lipid changes seen with these drugs (especially pioglitazone) might be beneficial. In small research studies these drugs have been shown to prevent the reblockage of coronary arteries after they have been opened with a procedure called coronary angioplasty. These medicines also seem to help fatty liver, an important abnormality found in many people with type 2 diabetes and which can lead to liver damage (cirrhosis of the liver).

Side Effects

The main side effects of these medicines are weight gain and fluid retention. The weight gain tends to be around the abdomen. Despite the weight gain, the glucose levels generally fall. Fluid retention can cause ankle swelling, and in individuals with heart disease these medicines can cause heart failure. (The symptoms of heart failure include swelling of the legs and shortness of breath on exertion.) The fluid retention is more of a problem if you are also on insulin. The FDA has emphasized that these drugs should not be used in people who are at risk for heart failure. A recent combined analysis of all people with type 2 diabetes who were in clinical trials with rosiglitazone for more than six months suggested that individuals on rosiglitazone had more heart attacks than those who were not taking the drug. This finding still requires confirmation. Pioglitazone, on the other hand, does not seem to have this effect. Very rarely, these medicines can cause swelling of the retina at the back of the eye and cause blurred vision. Stopping the medicine resolves this side effect. The first medicine in this class was called troglitazone (Rezulin) and was withdrawn from clinical use because it caused liver failure. This problem does not appear to occur with rosiglitazone and pioglitazone, but the FDA recommends that people with liver disease should not use this drug. If you are prescribed a medicine from this group, have your liver enzymes tested periodically, and if liver enzyme abnormalities develop, the medicine should be discontinued. In experimental animals, these drugs increase bone turnover, and there are preliminary reports that they may *increase the risk of fractures* in women but not men. Further studies are needed to confirm these findings.

EXENATIDE

How It Works

This medicine (see Table 6-5) lowers glucose levels by four different means:

- It acts on the beta cells to cause insulin release.
- It decreases the glucagon release from alpha cells after meals.
- It slows stomach emptying.
- It reduces appetite and promotes weight loss.

Exenatide works in exactly the same way as glucagon-like polypeptide 1 (GLP-1), a hormone released by the small intestine in response to food. GLP-1 is rapidly broken down in the body, and so would have to be given continuously to be effective. On the other hand, exenatide needs to be injected only twice a day, within one hour of breakfast and one hour of the evening meal. The recommended dose is 5 μg (micrograms) twice a day for the first month, and if well tolerated, it is increased to 10 μg twice a day.

Exenatide is particularly effective at releasing insulin when glucose is elevated, but not as effective when glucose is normal. This glucose-dependent insulin release means that there is less risk for hypoglycemia when this drug is used on its own. Backup supplies of exenatide should be stored in the refrigerator (not the freezer), but the pen you are currently using can be kept at room temperature.

In experimental animals and in islets in culture, exenatide has a protective effect preventing their death (apoptosis). This raises the possibility that if this is the case in humans (not yet shown), then this medicine may prevent loss of beta cells with time and may even reverse diabetes.

Table 6-5	Injectable Diabetes Medicine That Mimics the Effect of the Gut Hormone GLP-1		
Generic Drug Name (Brand Name in Parentheses)		**Strength**	**Daily Dose**
Incretins			
Exenatide (Byetta)		5 and 10 μg	Inject 5 μg within 1 hour of breakfast and dinner; increase to 10 μg twice a day after about a month; lasts for 6 hours

Note: μg = micrograms.

Side Effects

Nausea occurs in approximately 40 percent of individuals using exenatide. In approximately 5 percent of these people, the nausea is so severe that the drug has to be stopped. For most people, the nausea is manageable and tends to improve with time. Sometimes people tolerate the 5-μg dose but not the 10-μg dose. People who have gastroparesis should not use exenatide because it slows gastric emptying, making the symptoms of gastroparesis worse. Exenatide cannot be used if you have severe kidney failure.

SITAGLIPTIN

How It Works

Sitagliptin inhibits an enzyme (called dipeptidyl protease IV, DPP IV) and so prolongs the action of the hormone glucagon-like polypeptide 1 (GLP-1) that is released from the intestine in response to food. (See Table 6-6.) The prolonged activity of the released GLP-1 lowers glucose levels by three different means:

- It stimulates the release of insulin from beta cells.
- It inhibits glucagon release from alpha cells.
- It slows down stomach emptying.

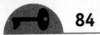

Table 6-6	Oral Diabetes Medicine That Prolongs the Activity of Gut Hormones Such as GLP-1 That Stimulate Insulin Release		
Generic Drug Name (Brand Name in Parentheses)		**Strength**	**Daily Dose**
DPP IV inhibitors (incretin enhancers)			
Sitagliptin (Januvia)		25, 50, and 100 mg	100 mg once a day is the normal dose; 25–50 mg is used if there is kidney failure; lasts 24 hours

The usual dose is 100 mg once a day and is reduced to 50 mg or 25 mg if there is kidney failure. In experimental animals, it seems to have a protective effect on beta cells. This has not yet been shown in humans. It does not cause hypoglycemia when used on its own. Sitagliptin does not reduce appetite and does not cause weight loss. Vildagliptin (Galvus), another DPP IV inhibitor, is likely to become available in the future.

Side Effects

The main side effects of sitagliptin appear to be a sore throat and headaches. There was also a small increase in the number of white blood cells (these are the cells that fight bacterial infections). It has only recently been approved for clinical use, so long-term safety data is lacking.

PRAMLINTIDE

How It Works

Pramlintide limits the glucose rise after meals by slowing stomach emptying and lowering the postmeal glucagon levels. (See Table 6-7.) It also causes modest weight loss: two to four pounds on average.

When beta cells release insulin, they also release another protein called islet amyloid polypeptide (IAPP or amylin). The normal function of IAPP is not well understood, but it may have a role in appetite regulation. Pramlintide is a modified form of IAPP. It is approved for use by people with type 2 diabetes who are using insulin and for people with type 1 diabetes. Pramlintide is given by injection just before a meal at the same time as the insulin.

Table 6-7	Injectable Diabetes Medicine That Mimics the Effects of a Beta Cell Protein Called Islet Amyloid Polypeptide	
Generic Drug Name (Brand Name in Parentheses)	**Strength**	**Daily Dose**
Pramlintide (Symlin)	5-ml vial containing 0.6 mg/ml	Type 2 patients on insulin: start at 60-μg dose 3 times a day (10 units on U100 insulin syringe); increase to 120 μg 3 times a day (20 units) if no nausea for 3 to 7 days. Give immediately before meal. For type 1 patients, start at 15 μg 3 times a day (2.5 units on U100 insulin syringe) and increase gradually to 60 μg (10 units) 3 times a day. Reduce the insulin by 50% when you start to avoid hypoglycemia.

Note: μg = micrograms.

Side Effects

The main side effect of Pramlintide is nausea and vomiting, especially in people who have gastroparesis.

DIABETES MEDICINE COMBINATIONS

Many people with diabetes are on more than one medicine to control glucose levels, and pharmaceutical companies make combination pills—that is, a pill containing two different diabetes medicines. Since many insurance companies make their customers pay a part of the cost of each prescription (a copayment), the combination pill has the benefit of eliminating one of the copayments. However, the disadvantage of these combinations is that you lose some of the flexibility of adjusting the individual doses of the medicines.

Also, if you need to discontinue one of the two medications, you may have to go back to the doctor and get a prescription for the single medicine that you are continuing. The combination pill usually has a different name, and often patients (and physicians) forget that the pill contains two different medicines. If you are prescribed a combination pill, make sure that you are not taking both a combination pill and one of the components of the combination pill as a separate pill. Table 6-8 is a summary of the different diabetes combination medicines that are currently available, with generic and brand names.

Table 6-8 Combination Drugs Currently Available for Type 2 Diabetes	
Brand Name	**Drug Combination**
Avandamet	Rosiglitazone with metformin
Avandryl	Rosiglitazone with glimepiride
Actoplus Met	Pioglitazone with metformin
Duetact	Pioglitazone with glimepiride
Glucovance	Glyburide with metformin
Metaglip	Glipizide with metformin
Janumet	Sitagliptin with metformin

Insulin

The goal of insulin therapy is to mimic the insulin secretion pattern that is seen in people without diabetes through the use of injections or an insulin pump. Normally there are two patterns of insulin release:

- Basal insulin, or background insulin, which is continuously released from the beta cells and regulates the glucose production from the liver

- Bolus insulin, which is insulin released in response to food and controls the glucose changes after meals

There are two types of insulin available for treating people with diabetes:

- Fast-acting insulin covers the glucose level rise in response to food
- Long-acting insulin provides the background insulin

Insulin preparations differ in how quickly they start working, when they have their peak effect, and how long they last. Table 6-9 summarizes the characteristics of the currently available insulin preparations.

FAST-ACTING INSULIN PREPARATIONS

There are four fast-acting insulin preparations:

- Regular insulin
- Insulin lispro
- Insulin aspart
- Insulin glulisine

Table 6-9   Characteristics of the Currently Available Insulins

Insulin Preparations	How Soon Does It Start Acting?	Peak Effect	How Long Does It Last?
Insulins lispro, aspart, glulisine	5–15 minutes	1–1.5 hours	3–4 hours
Human regular	30–60 minutes	2 hours	6–8 hours
Human NPH	2–4 hours	6–7 hours	10–20 hours
Insulin glargine	1.5 hours	Flat	About 24 hours
Insulin detemir	1 hour	Almost flat	17 hours

Regular Insulin

The following is true about regular insulin:

- Regular insulin has to be injected thirty minutes before a meal so that the insulin peak matches the glucose peak. However, this is inconvenient, and the advice is often ignored.

- After injection, the rise in insulin level is not as rapid as might be desirable to match the glucose rise.

- The duration of action is longer than desirable so that the insulin level remains a little high even after the glucose level has fallen, increasing the risk of hypoglycemia. Also, a larger dose of regular insulin lasts longer than a smaller dose.

- Rubbing or warming the injection site (for example, by sitting in a hot tub) speeds up insulin absorption.

- Insulin injected into the abdomen absorbs more rapidly than that injected in the upper arm, and absorption in the thigh is the slowest.

For these reasons, scientists have modified the insulin molecule to create **insulin analogs**, which have more desirable absorption properties after **subcutaneous injection**. The three fast-acting insulin analogs are:

- Insulin lispro (brand name Humalog)
- Insulin aspart (brand name Novolog)
- Insulin glulisine (brand name Apidra)

These insulins get absorbed more quickly after injection, so that they can be injected within fifteen minutes of starting a meal. After injection, the peak insulin is twice as high as after regular insulin, without a significant delay. The site of injection also has less of an impact: the abdomen, upper arm, and thighs all have relatively similar absorption. Since these fast-acting analogs are absorbed faster, their effect lasts for

The Technical Side of Regular Insulin

Regular insulin consists of aggregates of six molecules of insulin complexed to two zinc ions (a hexamer). After subcutaneous (under the skin) injection, the regular insulin hexamers become diluted by the tissue fluids and become monomers (single molecules), which then enter the circulation and have their effects.

a shorter period of time—about four hours (rather than six hours). These properties make these insulins more effective at controlling the glucose rise after meals. Clinical studies have shown that when these insulin analogs are used in an optimal manner, you can achieve improved glucose control with less risk of hypoglycemia.

However, there are some cautionary notes: first, because the peak level of the insulin with the analogs is higher after a meal, it is important for you to be more precise in counting the carbohydrates you are consuming. Regular insulin is more forgiving of errors in carbohydrate counting. Also, if you were to consume a very fatty meal, which delays glucose absorption, you have to inject these insulin analogs *after* a meal.

LONG-ACTING INSULIN PREPARATIONS

There are three long-acting insulin preparations:

- NPH insulin
- Insulin glargine (brand name Lantus)
- Insulin detemir (brand name Levemir)

Mixing regular insulin with a fish protein called protamine forms a crystal (neutral protamine Hagedorn, NPH), which dissolves slowly when injected subcutaneously, so that the effect on average lasts for about eight hours (shorter duration for very small doses and longer duration for large doses). The crystals of NPH insulin appear white to the naked eye, and they tend to settle in the insulin vial. This is why you should mix the NPH insulin (by rolling the bottle between the palms of your hands) before drawing it up in the syringe.

Insulin glargine is human insulin that is modified so that it is soluble in a more acidic solution. It looks clear in the bottle, and when injected it precipitates in the tissues and is then slowly released into the bloodstream. Since it is acidic, the manufacturer recommends it should be given as a separate injection and not mixed in the syringe with the regular or fast-acting insulin analogs. For most people, insulin glargine works for twenty-four hours. For some individuals (especially small children and small adults who take low doses of insulin), the effect does not last for twenty-four hours, and in these cases, doses have to be given twice a day.

Insulin detemir is a human insulin modified to have a fatty acid chain attached to it. This fatty acid chain binds to the blood protein albumin, and this complex acts as a storage form of insulin in the blood, with the insulin being slowly released for its effect, which lasts up to eighteen hours. It usually needs to be given twice a day to cover the twenty-four hours.

INSULIN TIPS

- All insulin vials have a concentration of 100 units of insulin in 1 ml and are therefore called U100 insulins. A more concentrated form of regular insulin called U500 insulin (that is, 500 units of insulin in 1 ml) is available for use by people who need extremely large amounts of insulin.

- You can keep the vials of insulin you are currently using at room temperature. Do not "cook" them in a hot car or leave them in the sun, as this will affect their efficacy.

- Any spare insulin vials, insulin cartridges, or disposable insulin pens you have should be kept in the refrigerator (not the freezer) and are good until the expiration date.

- Although insulins are very stable at room temperature, it is best to open a new bottle monthly. Experience has shown that sometimes they go bad.

- All insulins, with the exception of NPH, are clear liquids, so you do not have to mix them. When you mix NPH insulin, it is best to roll the bottle in the palm of your hand and *not* to shake it vigorously, because that will introduce bubbles and the dosing will be inaccurate.

- You can mix NPH insulin with regular insulin or the fast-acting insulin analogs in a syringe. However, mixing the long-acting insulin analogs (insulin glargine or detemir) with the fast-acting insulin analogs is not recommended. Most people no longer mix insulin: they give separate injections of the long-acting and fast-acting insulin analogs. If you mix regular or fast-acting insulin analogs and NPH insulin, just remember to draw the clear insulin before the cloudy insulin. You can ask a diabetes educator or your pharmacist to explain the mixing procedure to you.

- In the following sidebar you'll find all the premixed insulins that are currently available. They are often used by people with type 2 diabetes who take two injections a day: once before breakfast and once before dinner. They are available as various proportions of long-acting insulin with either regular or fast-acting insulin analog. Generally speaking, NPH and regular insulin mixtures (70/30 and 50/50 insulin) are being prescribed less and less. They have been replaced with long-acting insulin preparations and fast-acting insulin analog mixtures such as Humalog Mix 75/25 and Novolog Mix 70/30. These are popular because they can be injected immediately before a meal and they are much better at controlling the postmeal blood glucose rise.

- Before the introduction of insulin analogs in 1996, when regular insulin was a clear liquid and the long-acting insulin (NPH, Ultralente, and Lente) was cloudy, people had no problem remembering to take the clear insulin before meals and cloudy insulin before bedtime. Now, with both fast-acting and long-acting insulins being clear, it is easy to make a mistake and take the wrong insulin, increasing the risk for hypoglycemia. So, it is imperative that you read the labels on your vials of insulin. If you make a mistake and take a large amount of fast-acting insulin analog at bedtime, do not panic. Just check your blood glucose levels frequently and take additional carbohydrates for the next four to six hours until all the insulin has gone from your system. If you are having problems keeping your glucose level up, then go to the emergency room.

DID YOU KNOW?

Insulin Preparations Available in the United States

Short-Acting Insulins	**Long-Acting Insulins**
Regular insulin	NPH insulin
Insulin lispro (Humalog)	Insulin glargine (Lantus)
Insulin aspart (Novolog)	Insulin detemir (Levemir)
Insulin glulisine (Apidra)	

Premixed Insulins
70 percent NPH/30 percent regular (70/30 insulin)
50 percent NPH/50 percent regular (50/50 insulin)
75 percent NPL/25 percent insulin lispro (Humalog Mix 75/25)
50 percent NPL/50 percent insulin lispro (Humalog Mix 50/50)
70 percent insulin aspart protamine/30 percent insulin aspart (Novolog Mix 70/30)

Inhaled Insulin
Exubera (1 mg and 3 mg blister packets of powdered regular insulin)

DID YOU KNOW?

Exubera (Inhaled Insulin)

Inhaled insulin is not a new insulin: it is simply an old insulin (regular insulin) that is delivered into the body in a different way. You use an inhaler (very much like an asthma inhaler) to inhale the insulin powder, which is available in 1 mg and 3 mg blister packs.

The 1 mg pack is equivalent to 3 units of insulin, and the 3 mg pack is about 8 units of insulin. Three 1 mg inhalations are not equivalent to one 3 mg inhalation—you get one-third more insulin with the former. This is because three separate inhalations result in more insulin being absorbed than one larger-dose inhalation.

Only about 10 percent of the delivered dose gets into the circulation, so an average adult has to inhale 300 to 400 units of insulin a day. The inhaled insulin is rapidly absorbed—the insulin profile is very much like the injected fast-acting insulin analogs, except it lasts longer (up to six hours).

The biggest unanswered question about inhaled insulin is whether it will damage the lungs if used for a long time. The studies so far have shown that when someone starts using inhaled insulin, there is a small negative effect on the lung function, but then these lung changes stabilize and do not get worse with time. Therefore, the FDA requires that anyone taking inhaled insulin should have lung function tests before starting it, at six months, and then yearly.

You should not use Exubera if you have lung disease such as asthma or bronchitis, or if you are a smoker. Smoking results in more of the insulin being absorbed, and you have to stop smoking for at least six months before you can start on inhaled insulin. There are higher levels of antibodies to insulin in the blood after using inhaled insulin compared to injected insulin, but this does not seem to have a negative effect. Other side effects include cough, shortness of breath, sore throat, and dry mouth. In the clinical trials of Exubera, approximately 2,500 adult patients with type 1 and type 2 diabetes were studied for an average duration of about two years. Many more people will need to take inhaled insulin for longer periods before we can be sure that it is as safe as injected insulin.

USING AN INSULIN PUMP

An insulin pump is a device the size of a pager. It contains a syringe or reservoir filled with a *fast-acting insulin*, a battery-powered syringe plunger, and a small computer to control the insulin delivery. The syringe is attached to tubing, which in turn is attached to a small plastic tube (cannula) inserted under the skin (see Figure 6-1). The pump can be programmed to put tiny drops of insulin into the subcutane-

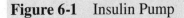

Figure 6-1   Insulin Pump

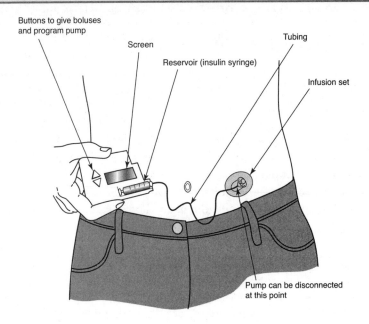

Buttons to give boluses
and program pump

Screen

Reservoir (insulin syringe)

Tubing

Infusion set

Pump can be disconnected
at this point

ous tissues every three to ten minutes day and night—this is the basal insulin. When you eat, you can program the pump to give a bolus of insulin for the food. Thus, when you are on the pump, you use only a fast-acting insulin to provide both your basal and bolus needs.

Often, people with type 1 diabetes will decide to go on an insulin pump for their diabetes control. The pump does not check glucose levels, nor does it decide how much insulin to give. It does allow you to tailor your basal insulin to your needs. With a pump, you are better able to reduce your insulin levels for exercise. A major advantage is that the pump reduces the number of insulin injections—essentially, you are doing one injection every three days.

There is a fair amount of work involved in using an insulin pump, and you will have to be proactive in terms of managing the diabetes and feel comfortable taking the initiative and adjusting your insulin dose for food and activity. You will need to check your blood glucose as many times or more often than when you were on injections. You also have to set basal rates and make decisions on how much bolus insulin you should give. Table 6-10 summarizes the advantages and disadvantages of insulin pumps.

Table 6-10 Advantages and Disadvantages of Insulin Pump Therapy (Also Known as CSII—Continuous Subcutaneous Insulin Infusion)	
Advantages of Pumps	**Disadvantages of Pumps**
One injection every three days	Being attached to a machine
More precise basal insulin levels—especially overnight and first thing in the morning	No significant subcutaneous insulin reservoir—if the pump fails or infusion set kinks and you are not aware, you can go into ketoacidosis
Adjust basal insulin levels for exercise	
More precise boluses—adjust by 0.05-unit increments	Increased risk of skin abscess
	Expense
Insulin on board feature—which reminds user that previous insulin bolus is still active— helps avoid stacking of insulin boluses	

Is the Insulin Pump Right for You?

Before you go to a pump clinic (which your physician will recommend), you should already have these self-management skills:

- Be on a basal-bolus insulin regimen
- Counting carbohydrates (see Chapter 8)
- Know how to adjust food and insulin for exercise (see Chapter 9)
- Monitoring blood glucose levels frequently (see Chapter 5)
- Keeping written records (see Chapter 5)

The staff at the pump clinic will first explain what the pump can and cannot do. They will show you a pump, the tubing, and an insulin infusion cannula and explain how it is kept in place. They will answer questions about how a pump will impact your daily activities, such as sleeping, exercising, showering, and having sex. They will give you brochures about the pumps available from different manufacturers, explain the costs associated with pump therapy, and help fill out the paperwork for getting your insurance to pay for a pump. The pump team will also assess your self-management skills and make sure that they are optimal.

Choosing Your Infusion Set

The infusion set is the tiny plastic tube or cannula that you insert into the subcutaneous tissue. There are many different infusion sets available, and your pump educator will work with you to choose a set that will work best for you. There are some pump sets that have a cannula (plastic tubing) angled at 30 to 45 degrees, and some sets with a straight cannula (90 degrees). Most are made of Teflon, but there are some that are made of metal. The angled sets are more reliable than the straight sets in that they are less likely to get kinked, but the disadvantage of the angled sets is that the introducer needle is longer. Some sets need to be inserted manually, and others can be inserted with a spring-loaded insertion device. The insertion device makes it easier to place the sets in hard-to-reach places such as the buttocks. Inserting sets is clearly a little more painful than using a needle, but you are only doing it once every three days. For children, using a numbing lidocaine cream like EMLA or LMX 4 percent before insertion can make it easier.

Choosing Your Pump

The pumps that are available are all reliable and relatively easy to use. The companies that make insulin pump are Animas, Deltec, Medtronic MiniMed, Roche, and Insulet (OmniPod). The pumps do have some differences, and you may want to compare them to see what will work best for you (see Resources).

When comparing, you need to consider these features:

- The size of the reservoir—this is important if you are a large person and need higher doses of insulin
- How quickly the bolus is given
- The frequency of basal delivery
- How easy is it to program
- The type of service offered by the manufacturer. Pumps are complex and do malfunction. Your pump educators can advise you about their experiences with the various manufacturers.

If you call the representatives of the pump companies, they will meet you to demonstrate their products. The initial cost of the pump and related supplies is about $5,500. Once you have decided on a pump, the representative and your medical team will help fill out the forms to get approval from your health insurer.

Setting Up Your Insulin Pump

Once your pump is approved, the manufacturer will ship it to your house. A pump educator from the manufacturer (also paid for by the manufacturer) will come to your house and explain the features of the pump and how to program it. He will also show you how to fill a reservoir without getting bubbles and how to prime the tubing. An inch of bubble in your tubing is equivalent to half a unit of insulin. Thus, having bubbles in your tubing can reduce the amount of insulin you are getting and can lead to high glucose levels. Once the tubing is primed, you can insert the infusion set and attach the tubing. A 0.3- to 1.0-unit bolus may be needed to fill the "dead space" in the infusion set. The pump trainer should teach you how to use a pump using saline (salt water, as opposed to insulin). Ideally, you should do this for about a week before your planned initiation of insulin in the pump. During this time, you can practice changing sets, filling reservoirs, priming tubes, and adjusting basal and bolus doses.

It is very important to use a clean technique when placing the infusion set in order to avoid infections. Usually you should change the infusion set immediately after a shower. If you change it at other times, wash your hands thoroughly and wipe a two-inch-diameter area of skin with IV prep, Hibiclens, or Betadine skin swabs. Let the skin dry naturally—do not blow air on it. Make sure that you use a sterile infusion set—that is, one that has not been previously opened. For many patients, the adhesive patch that is included as a part of the infusion set is sufficient to keep it in place. People who are very active or who tend to sweat a lot should first apply a bio-occlusive dressing such as IV 3000 on the skin and then insert the infusion set through the dressing.

The abdomen is the preferred site for the infusion sets. Other sites that can be used are the buttocks, hips, outer thighs, or the backs of arms. You should avoid areas with scar tissue, tattoos, visible blood vessels, and pierced areas. Move at least two inches from the previous site, and avoid using the same site again for seven to ten days. If your site looks infected—for example, if you have red spots, pain, or swelling, then you must contact your medical team early, so any infection can be treated. The sets are changed every three days.

Starting Pump Therapy

You will meet your pump care team a few weeks before pump start, and they will work with you to decide what basals and boluses you should start with. Usually, you need less insulin than you are taking by injection, perhaps 80 percent as much.

For example, if you were on 20 units of insulin glargine, 80 percent of this would be 16 units. Dividing this by 24 hours gives you 0.67 units per hour. You would probably start at even a lower dose, and the initial basals might be

- Midnight—0.45 units per hour

- 3 A.M.—0.5 units per hour

- 9 A.M.—0.45 units per hour

Usually, as illustrated in this example, more insulin is needed very early in the morning because of the normal hormonal changes in the body that occur at that time (referred to as the **dawn phenomenon**). The bolus insulin ratios are usually the same as with the injections—for example 1 unit per 15 grams carbohydrate and 1 unit for 50 mg/dl over target.

Living with the Pump

The pump will deliver basal insulin into the subcutaneous tissue at the rate you program throughout the day and night. When you want to give a correction insulin dose or insulin for food, you instruct the pump by pressing some buttons. Here are some other issues that come up with the pump:

- Usually the pump infusion set, reservoir, and tubing are changed every three days. The reservoirs hold 200 to 300 units of insulin, which for most people is more than enough for three days' use.

- When you sleep, you can put the pump under your pillow or in your pajama pocket.

- You can keep the pump on or take it off when exercising (see Chapter 9).

- The pumps are water resistant, and some are waterproof. Most people take off the pump for showers or for swimming.

- Things that can go wrong include air in the tubing and kinks in the cannula. Both of these problems will result in high glucose levels. As you get more experience with using pumps and infusion sets, these problems happen less and less.

- The pumps use AA or AAA batteries. There are alarms to alert you when the battery runs low.

Nutritional Supplements That Lower Glucose Levels

When considering nutritional supplements to lower glucose levels, you need to keep a number of issues in mind:

- There is limited information supporting the glucose-lowering effect of many supplements. Sometimes there are just a few anecdotal reports rather than carefully performed scientific studies. What scientific studies there are, on closer inspection, have major flaws. The reason there are no large clinical studies for supplements is that these studies are very expensive to do. In some cases, the evidence that a particular chemical may have a role in glucose control is based on experiments in animals with a severe deficiency of the chemical. But this type of deficiency may occur only infrequently in humans. For example, chromium deficiency in rats causes insulin resistance, but it is difficult to show that degree of deficiency in

DID YOU KNOW?

The Cure for Type 1 Diabetes

A pancreas transplant will cure type 1 diabetes. So why doesn't everyone with type 1 diabetes get a pancreas transplant? There are two reasons. First, there are only a limited number of donor pancreata available—a few thousand—whereas there are about a million people with type 1 diabetes. Second, people who get an organ transplant have to be on medicines to prevent the body's immune system from attacking and rejecting the organ. These immunosuppressive medicines have serious side effects, such as making the individual more susceptible to infections and increasing the risk of developing a cancer in the future. You are likely to be offered a pancreas transplant if you have kidney failure and you are on a list for a donor kidney. Because getting two organs simultaneously has additional risks, some restrictions do apply. For example, if you have a history of heart attacks or strokes, you may not be a candidate for simultaneous pancreas-kidney transplant. A pancreas transplant alone—that is, getting a donor pancreas when you have normal kidney function—is also occasionally done. You may be a candidate for this if you continue to have frequent severe hypoglycemic reactions despite all efforts by you and your medical team to prevent them, or if you have life-threatening complications due to uncontrolled diabetes.

Islet transplantation is currently an experimental procedure that can also cure type 1 diabetes. In islet transplantation, instead of transplanting the whole pancreas, the islets that make the insulin are isolated from the pancreas and injected into the blood vessel that supplies the liver. The islets lodge in the liver and work normally, releasing insulin in response to changes in glucose levels. Islet transplantation is a much simpler procedure compared to pancreas transplantation. It is done in the x-ray department of a hospital rather than in an operating room. Also, if islet transplantation proves successful in curing both type 1 *and* type 2 diabetes permanently, there is the possibility of creating islets in a test tube from stem cells, making the treatment available for many more people with diabetes. Currently, with few exceptions, the "cure" seems to be temporary, with islet function declining with time so that most people need to go back on insulin after a couple of years. This may change in the future as we better understand the factors that cause the islets to fail. People who get an islet transplant have to take antirejection medicines, and therefore researchers restrict this procedure to people who have a history of frequent severe hypoglycemic reactions or complications due to uncontrolled diabetes.

humans consuming a normal diet, and so the relevance to human diabetes is unclear.

• Since nutritional supplements are not regulated in the same manner as pharmaceutical medicines, supplements may vary in terms of potency.

• Just because a compound is not regulated and is natural does not make it safe—there could be serious side effects, and the supplement could also affect the metabolism of other drugs that are taken at the same time.

In 2003, the ADA published a review of thirty-six different herbs and nine vitamin/mineral supplements used for glucose control in diabetes. The reader is directed to this review for further information (see Resources). I will briefly discuss here some of the more popular supplements.

CINNAMON

In a laboratory cell culture, extracts of cinnamon have been shown to enhance the action of insulin. In 2003, the journal *Diabetes Care* published a study that reported that cinnamon extract lowered fasting glucose, triglycerides, and LDL cholesterol in thirty patients with type 2 diabetes. This study got a lot of attention in the media, and many people with diabetes wonder if cinnamon would help their diabetes. However, a smaller study published in *The Journal of Nutrition* in 2006 with twelve subjects taking cinnamon extract did not show any benefit. In both studies the patients were also on other diabetes medicine. In the 2003 study they were all on sulfonylureas, whereas in the 2006 study they were on sulfonylureas with or without metformin or metformin or thiazolidinediones with or without metformin or a reduced-calorie diet. It is possible that this difference may explain the lack of response in the second study.

CHROMIUM

When rats are given a diet deficient in chromium, they have higher glucose levels. Similarly, humans who are on intravenous nutrition (total parenteral nutrition), if they are not given chromium supplements, have higher glucose levels and insulin resistance. It has not been shown that people with diabetes have chromium deficiency, but when chromium picolinate has been given to people with diabetes, a number of studies have shown a benefit. For example, in a study published in the journal *Diabetes Care* in 2006, seventeen patients with type 2 diabetes on sulfonylureas who were given 1,000 micrograms of chromium had an improvement in glucose control and insulin sensitivity. This dose is much higher than the recommended daily dose, which is 20 to 35 micrograms daily. It appears to be fairly safe at the high dose, although there have been two cases of kidney problems and one case of liver damage reported. A longer-duration study with a larger number of subjects is needed to find out if chromium supplements are beneficial for people with diabetes. An important question is whether the supplement adds much for patients who already may be on several drugs for their diabetes.

SELENIUM

The trace element selenium is important in the activity of a number proteins in the body—these are known as selenoproteins. Glutathione peroxidases and cellular antioxidants are selenoproteins, and so selenium's antioxidant properties have been a focus of clinical studies. So far, however, there are no studies showing that selenium supplementation is beneficial in people with diabetes.

PANAX QUINQUEFOLIUS (AMERICAN GINSENG)

Several small studies reported an improvement in fasting glucose and HbA1c with 3 grams of American ginseng. The studies are of limited duration (eight weeks). Reported side effects of American ginseng include insomnia, high blood pressure, and anxiety.

The ADA review found that there was inadequate evidence to support use of herbal medicine or mineral supplements in the treatment of diabetes. If you decide to use them, buy your supplements from reputable suppliers—those with USP (United States Pharmacopeia) or NF (National Formulary) labels are preferred (see Resources). The National Nutritional Foods Association good-manufacturing practices (NNFA GMP) and ConsumerLab.com also test the quality of herbal and dietary supplements.

Summary

- If you have type 2 diabetes, your treatment will involve:
  - Oral medicine:
    - Those that stimulate the beta cells to produce insulin (sulfonylureas, meglitinides, and D-phenylalanine derivatives)
    - Those that regulate glucose production in the liver (biguanides, such as metformin)
    - Those that slow the breakdown of starches (alpha-glucosidase inhibitors such as acarbose and miglitol)
    - Those that sensitize the tissues to the effects of insulin (insulin sensitizers) such as rosiglitazone and pioglitazone

- Those that inhibit DPP-IV (the gliptins or incretin enhancers), for example, sitagliptin and vildagliptin
- Injected medicine:
  - Exenatide, an incretin mimic, stimulates insulin release.
  - Pramlintide (Amylin) slows stomach emptying and lowers glucagon levels.
  - Insulin—all the currently available insulins are human insulins. They differ in the onset and duration of action. The newer fast-acting insulin analogs (lispro, aspart, and glulisine) and the two long-acting insulin analogs (glargine and detemir) have better absorption characteristics after subcutaneous injection, allowing for better regulation of glucose levels with less risk of hypoglycemia.
- If you have type 1 diabetes, you will need to replace the insulin that the body no longer makes by using insulin injections or an insulin pump.
- If you have good diabetes self-management skills, an insulin pump offers a number of advantages:
  - Fewer injections (one injection every three days)
  - Better dosing of basal insulin for your needs
  - Easier adjustment of insulin doses for exercise

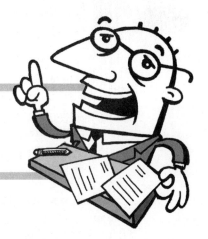

CHAPTER 7

Hypoglycemia (Low Glucose Reaction)

Hypoglycemia is low glucose reaction—other names for it include **insulin reaction**, insulin shock, or "a low." This chapter gives you all the details of this condition.

What Does Hypoglycemia Feel Like?

The first time a person with diabetes gets a low glucose reaction—usually at a glucose level of about 54 mg/dl, he or she usually gets shaky, sweaty, and hungry. Other symptoms include anxiety and nausea. These are very much like the symptoms you get when you are extremely nervous and are called **autonomic symptoms**. It's your body's way of telling you that your glucose is low and you should eat. If these autonomic symptoms are ignored, the glucose levels fall into a range where the brain is starved of energy (around glucose value of 49 mg/dl) and you feel irritable, you can't think clearly, your vision is blurred, you feel tired, you have a headache, and you have difficulty speaking. These are called **neuroglycopenic symp-**

toms. When the symptoms are severe, they can prevent you from treating the low glucose levels, and if the glucose level falls even further, into the less-than-30 range, you can lose consciousness or even have a seizure. Table 7-1 gives typical symptoms of hypoglycemia.

If you have had diabetes a very long time and/or have had several recent low glucose reactions, you may not get the autonomic symptoms, or they may occur at lower glucose levels. So often the first indication that your glucose is low may be neuroglycopenic symptoms such as feeling tired or having blurred vision. Occasionally patients will tell me that they had a glucose measurement in the 30s and they felt fine. This inability to recognize hypoglycemia until the levels are very low is known as **hypoglycemic unawareness**, and it is of concern because the glucose levels only have to fall a little further before there is loss of consciousness.

What Should My Glucose Levels Be?

In people without diabetes, glucose values can be in the 60 to 70 mg/dl range or even lower with prolonged fasting. The problem with diabetes is that if you are taking medicines that can cause hypoglycemia, like insulin and sulfonylureas, a glucose level around 60 is of concern because it could go down even further. The ADA defines a glucose level of 70 mg/dl or less as hypoglycemia, even if you feel fine and show no symptoms. Thus, if you are on medicines that can cause hypoglycemia, you should take action if the glucose level is below 70. If, however, you are controlling your diabetes with diet only, then values in the 60 to 80 range are fine and do not need treatment.

Table 7-1 Typical Hypoglycemic Symptoms	
Autonomic Symptoms (due to the activation of the sympathetic nervous system)	**Neuroglycopenic Symptoms (due to the brain being starved of glucose)**
Sweating	Drowsiness
Shaking	Confusion
Anxiety	Slurred speech
Racing heart	Blurred vision
	Tiredness
	Irritability

One thing to be aware of is that if your glucose has been running high for a while, you may get the symptoms of low glucose even when the glucose level is in the normal range—such as 100 mg/dl. As your diabetes control improves, this will change so that the symptoms will appear only with lower glucose levels.

What Causes Hypoglycemia?

Hypoglycemia in people with diabetes is a consequence of three things: behavioral issues, impaired counterregulatory systems, and complications of diabetes.

BEHAVIORAL ISSUES

Behavioral issues include overestimating carbohydrate intake, failing to adjust insulin for exercise, and stacking of insulin and overaggressive treatment of high glucose levels.

Overestimation of Carbohydrate Intake

One of the most common reasons for recurrent hypoglycemia is injecting too much insulin or taking too much oral medication for the amount of carbohydrates ingested. You may overestimate the amount of carbohydrate in the food or eat less than planned, or you may be delayed in eating after taking the insulin or medicine. For example, a number of times, I have had patients inject a dose of insulin in the car before they went to a restaurant. At the restaurant, the food did not come at the expected time, and so their glucose level went low. Another example is when patients are asked to fast for a lab test (such as a lipid profile): they do not realize that they should delay taking their insulin or diabetic medicine until after the test. Drinking alcohol in excess (see Chapter 8), especially on an empty stomach, can also cause hypoglycemia.

Failure to Adjust for Exercise

In Chapter 9, I explain why people with diabetes, especially type 1 diabetes, can find glucose control with exercise particularly challenging. Hypoglycemia can occur during or even several hours after exercise, and so glucose levels need to be monitored and food and insulin adjusted. Failure to do this can lead to hypoglycemia. Unexpected exercise can also be a challenge: I remember seeing a sixty-eight-year-old woman with type 1 diabetes in my office, and during her visit the fire alarm went off, and so I escorted her down six sets of stairs. When we sat down outside the building, I asked her to check her sugar, even though she felt fine. She was surprised to find that the glucose was down to 45 mg/dl!

"Stacking" Insulin and Overaggressive Treatment of High Glucose Levels

Some people with diabetes do not like their glucose levels to be high, and they treat every high glucose level aggressively. These individuals who "stack" their insulin—that is, give another dose of insulin before the first injection has had its full action—can leave themselves open to hypoglycemia. A common mistake is to give insulin before a meal and then check the glucose level again an hour or two later and give additional insulin without realizing that the premeal insulin is still getting absorbed. To protect against stacking, the new insulin pumps have an "insulin-on-board" feature that keeps track of when the last insulin bolus was given and will remind the user that some of the previous insulin bolus is still getting absorbed if they attempt to give additional insulin.

FAILURE OF COUNTERREGULATORY SYSTEMS

Counterregulatory systems are those systems of the body—hormones and the nervous system—that are activated in response to falling glucose levels. In people with long-standing diabetes, some of the counterregulatory systems may not work as effectively, and this impairs the body's ability to respond adequately to falling glucose levels.

Lack of Glucagon Response

In new onset diabetes, glucagon levels rise in response to a falling glucose level, and this is the most important factor preventing a further fall in the glucose level. People with diabetes longer than five years lose this glucagon response. As a result, these individuals are at a significant disadvantage in protecting themselves against falling glucose levels. People who have diabetes because of pancreatitis or pancreatic surgery also lack glucagon and so are at increased risk for hypoglycemia.

Deficiency in Adrenaline and Noradrenaline Responses

Once the glucagon response is lost, the release of adrenaline and noradrenaline from the adrenal glands takes on added importance, alerting you to the falling glucose by causing your heart to race and making you shake. The adrenaline and noradrenaline responses are not as strong in people who have hypoglycemic unawareness due to repeated low glucose levels.

Cortisol Deficiency

The adrenal gland releases cortisol, a counterregulatory hormone that raises glucose. A deficiency of cortisol can increase the risk of hypoglycemia. Occasionally, people with type 1 diabetes can develop adrenal failure (Addison's disease). When this happens, their insulin requirements fall significantly, and unless their insulin dose is cut back, they will get hypoglycemic.

DIABETES COMPLICATIONS

Complications of diabetes include autonomic neuropathy, gastroparesis, and kidney failure.

Autonomic Neuropathy

The sympathetic nervous system is an important counterregulatory system that alerts a person that his or her glucose level is falling by causing symptoms such as shaking, a racing heart, and sweating. Failure of this system increases the risk of hypoglycemia.

Gastroparesis

Damage to the nerves to the stomach (gastroparesis) can delay food emptying, and if the insulin has been given before the meal, the peak of insulin action may occur before the food is absorbed, causing hypoglycemia.

Kidney Failure

People with diabetes who have kidney failure are at higher risk of hypoglycemia. There are several reasons for this. First, in kidney failure, the injected insulin and some of the oral diabetes medicines stay in the body for longer than normal. Second, people with kidney failure may have poor appetite and can get malnourished. The decreased fat and muscle mass due to malnutrition can impair the ability of the liver to produce glucose.

Treating Hypoglycemia

Treating hypoglycemia is fairly straightforward: eat or drink any food that has a lot of glucose and is easily absorbed. Sources of glucose include glucose tablets and gels that you can buy at your pharmacy. Fruit juice and nonfat milk are also good sources. Foods with a lot of fat such as chocolate are not as good because the fat will delay the absorption of the glucose. Fructose does not raise the blood glucose, but most foods that have fructose, such as honey and fruits, also have a lot of glucose.

Most times about 15 grams of carbohydrate is sufficient—but if your glucose is below 50 mg/dl, then 30 grams might be more appropriate. You should check your blood glucose fifteen minutes afterward, and if the glucose is still low take another 15 grams of carbohydrate and check the levels again in another fifteen to twenty minutes. Keep doing this until the glucose is in the safe range. It is important not to overdo your ingestion of carbohydrates because the glucose levels then go very high. In most people, 15 grams of glucose will raise the blood glucose level by about 40 mg/dl.

After your hypoglycemia has been treated satisfactorily, you may want to troubleshoot. Think about why it happened and what you can do to avoid a similar situation in the future: Does you insulin dose need to be adjusted? Do you need advice from your medical team?

GLUCAGON INJECTION

Injection of glucagon causes release of glucose from glycogen stores in the liver. If you are on insulin, keep an emergency glucagon kit at home and at work. Family members and colleagues at work should be educated about low glucose reactions and trained to inject glucagon in case you become very confused or lose consciousness due to hypoglycemia. You do not want to find out after the event that no one knew where the glucagon was kept and no one felt comfortable giving an injection.

A glucagon kit has a vial with 1 mg of powdered glucagon and a syringe containing diluting solution. To prepare the glucagon, inject all of the solution in the syringe into the vial of glucagon. Shake the vial to dissolve the glucagon and draw the solution back up into the syringe. Inject into the thigh, buttock, or arm. Glucagon injection works faster if it is injected into a muscle. For children who weigh less than forty-four pounds, inject half the contents of the glucagon syringe. Glucagon can cause nausea, and so the person being treated should be put on her side in case she vomits. The glucose level does not stay up for very long, and so once the person is awake, give her additional glucose by mouth. Using glucagon can allow the patient to be treated at home and avoid having to be admitted to the hospital, but paramedics should be called if the patient is having a seizure or is not responding within ten to fifteen minutes after the glucagon injection. If you know that the coma in the

person you are treating is due to sulfonylureas, do not give glucagon, becau
these circumstances glucagon can paradoxically cause a fall in glucose levels.

Preventing Hypoglyc

As you aim to get HbA1c levels (see Chapter 5) close to normal, the risk of hypoglycemia goes up. You can take the following measures to limit the risk:

- Set realistic targets—aim to keep premeal glucose levels between 90 and
  130 rather than at 80. Also, if you have recently had a severe hypoglycemic
  reaction, then for about six weeks aim to keep your glucose around 150.
  This will help you recover your ability to sense hypoglycemia to some
  degree.

- Learn to count carbohydrates and adjust insulin appropriately.

- Recognize behaviors that increase the risk of hypoglycemia and take steps
  to avoid them—for example, adjust the insulin for exercise, and drink
  alcohol in moderation and with food.

- Monitor blood glucose levels frequently, especially if you have type 1
  diabetes. You cannot achieve optimal glucose control with two or three
  checks a day. For tight control, check your blood glucose levels eight
  to twelve times a day (before meals and snacks, at bedtime, at 2 A.M.,
  before and after exercise, before driving, and when you have symptoms of
  hypoglycemia). Continuous glucose monitoring systems (see Chapter 5)
  can be set to give you a warning when glucose falls below the lower target
  set point.

- Pay attention to your symptoms of hypoglycemia. When you are busy, the
  temptation is to ignore the symptoms.

The University of Virginia has developed a training program called Blood Glucose Awareness Training (BGAT) for adults with type 1 diabetes to help them recognize, anticipate, and prevent extreme fluctuations in blood glucose levels. People
using this system have had fewer episodes of severe hypoglycemia and motor vehicle violations (see Resources).

Complications of Hypoglycemia

Hypoglycemia has some additional complications, which I discuss in the following
sections.

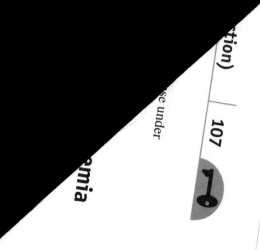

IA

...tion is uncomfortable—patients often tell me that it
...auses anxiety, and some people become so fearful that
...in than they need and keep glucose levels deliberately
...able reaction, and if this is happening to you, work with
...r your glucose targets. It may also be helpful to use a con-
...g system.

...ion of hypoglycemia is that it might put the person who is
hypoglyce...... ...le around him in danger—for example, if he is operating
machinery or driving. If the hypoglycemia is severe, the person can have a seizure,
weakness on one side of the body, or vision problems.

EFFECT ON INTELLECTUAL FUNCTION

Do repeated low glucose levels affect intellectual function? Research studies that
looked at this topic have not given clear answers. Part of the problem is that many
subjects who have severe hypoglycemic reactions also have other complications
from the diabetes that could impact intellectual function. What is reassuring is that
in the DCCT (a big research study of type 1 diabetes), severe hypoglycemic episodes did not result in decreased intellectual function over eighteen years of follow-
up. This, however, may not be true in very young children (less than five years old),
and for this group glucose levels should not be as tightly controlled as in adults (see
Chapter 14).

Driving and Hypoglycemia

Some of the medicines used to treat diabetes (insulin, sulfonylureas, repaglinide,
and nateglinide) can cause hypoglycemia, which can affect reflexes and judgment.
In addition, long-term diabetes complications, especially vision problems and neuropathy, may interfere with driving ability.

There have been a number of research studies that have looked at the impact of
diabetes on car accidents. Generally speaking, the impact appears to be modest if it
exists at all. It does seem that the risk for future car accidents is increased if there
has been a recent episode of severe hypoglycemia, hypoglycemic unawareness, or a
history of past crashes.

All the states have special licensing rules. The ADA website has information about your state (see Resources). Many states do not allow drivers who are on insulin to drive a commercial vehicle. Unfortunately, sometimes this means that some drivers are reluctant to go on insulin and have long-term poor glucose control.

Recommendations for safe driving if you have diabetes include the following:

- Check your blood glucose immediately before driving.
- Keep a glucose meter and fast-acting carbohydrates in the car.
- If you feel that your glucose levels are low, pull over and check.
- Be extra vigilant if you have complications, especially vision problems and diabetic neuropathy.

Summary

- Hypoglycemia, or low glucose reactions, can occur in people with both type 1 diabetes and type 2 diabetes.
- The autonomic symptoms of shaking, sweating, anxiety, and racing heart occur at a glucose level of around 54 mg/dl. If the glucose falls to around 49 mg/dl, the brain is starved of energy and you may feel tired or confused or have blurred vision (neurogenic symptoms). If the glucose falls even further into the 30s you can become comatose or have seizures.
- Hypoglycemia occurs principally because of
  - Overestimation of carbohydrate intake, failure to adjust insulin for exercise, or being overaggressive with insulin dosing
  - Impairment of the counterregulatory mechanisms, especially glucagon with long-standing diabetes
- To prevent hypoglycemia:
  - Be vigilant for symptoms of hypoglycemia
  - Monitor blood glucose levels frequently, especially before driving
  - Set realistic targets for your glucose: premeal targets between 90 and 130 mg/dl
- Treat hypoglycemic reactions with fast-acting carbohydrates such as juice or glucose tablets. Family members and colleagues should know how to use glucagon injections in an emergency.

CHAPTER 8

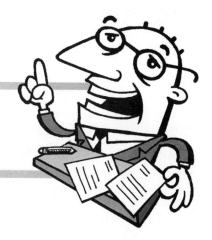

Diabetes and Nutrition

Nutrition has always played a central role in the treatment of diabetes. Before the discovery of insulin, people with type 1 diabetes could be kept alive for a few months by severely restricting carbohydrate intake and eating mostly fats and protein (a ketogenic diet). After the discovery of insulin in 1921, patients were able to eat more carbohydrates. However, the lack of home glucose monitoring and fast-acting insulins meant that there still were significant dietary restrictions. People with diabetes had to restrict carbohydrates and spread them throughout the day by eating three meals and three snacks. With the use of the new insulins analogs and blood glucose monitoring systems, the dietary restrictions are much less of a problem, but there are still some limitations, which I discuss in this chapter.

First, let me make some general points about diet in diabetes:

- There is no such thing as a diabetic diet. In fact, the diet for most people with diabetes is the same as the diet for people without diabetes. If you have diabetes, you do not have to buy foods specifically marketed to people with diabetes (for example, cookies, jams, and candy for people with diabetes, labeled as sugar-free).

• Obesity increases insulin resistance and insulin requirements, and so weight loss can significantly improve glucose control in people with type 2 diabetes. Weigh-loss strategies are generally the same as those for people without diabetes.

• Complications of diabetes such as gastroparesis (see Chapter 3), renal disease, and heart disease may require some additional dietary modifications.

The Three Components of a Meal

All foods are composed of three components—carbohydrates, fats, and proteins (also called macronutrients)—in varying amounts and quality. In the following sections I briefly discuss these three components as they pertain to diabetes.

CARBOHYDRATES (CHO)

Starchy foods such as rice, pasta, potatoes, breads, and beans and sugary foods like fruits and milk are rich in **carbohydrates (CHO)**. A focus on carbohydrates is necessary because the blood glucose rise after a meal is mostly due to the digestion and absorption of the carbohydrates in the meal. If you have type 1 diabetes, your insulin dosage for a meal is calculated according to the amount of carbohydrate in your meal.

If you have type 2 diabetes, you will need to have some carbohydrate restriction to avoid excessive increases in glucose levels after a meal, even if your diabetes is controlled with diet or oral medications.

The Glycemic Index

Different carbohydrates behave differently in the body: they vary in how much they raise the blood glucose level after ingestion. The **glycemic index** is the ranking given to carbohydrate-containing foods according to how much they raise blood glucose levels when compared to drinking 50 grams of glucose. For example, the rise in glucose levels after eating white bread is very similar to the rise after drinking glucose, so it has a glycemic index of 100 percent. In contrast, an apple has a glycemic index of 38, meaning that it will raise the glucose level much less.

The glycemic index depends on

• The fiber content of a food—the higher the fiber content, the lower the glycemic index.

- How much the food has been processed—so mashed potatoes have a higher glycemic index than baked potatoes, which are less processed. Similarly, al dente pasta has a lower glycemic index than overcooked pasta.

- The fat content of a food—fat delays stomach emptying and slows glucose absorption. Thus full-fat milk has a low glycemic index (27 percent).

When choosing what carbohydrates to eat, you cannot just focus on the glycemic index of each food, because the glycemic index of a food is affected by how much it has been processed and cooked, as well as the fat content of the meal. Instead, you want to eat fewer processed foods and more foods with high fiber, because these foods have a relatively low glycemic index. Table 8-1 lists some foods with low and high glycemic indexes. You can also go on the Internet to get a complete list of glycemic indexes of different foods (see Resources).

Fiber

Fibers are starches that are resistant to digestion (although approximately 10 percent of them are digested by bowel bacteria and absorbed). Soluble (or gel forming) fibers are found in apples and other fruits, and insoluble fibers are found in cereals and vegetables. For a person who has diabetes, foods with a high fiber content are beneficial because the fiber slows down glucose absorption and prevents high glucose levels after meals. There are two drugs, acarbose (Precose) and miglitol (Glyset), used in the treatment of type 2 diabetes that act by delaying the absorption of glucose from the bowel, so in a sense they act similarly to a high-fiber diet.

Table 8-1 Example of Glycemic Index	
Low Glycemic Index Foods (Under 55)	**High Glycemic Index Foods (Over 70)**
Apple	Bagel
Sweet potato	White bread
Lentils	French baguette
Kidney beans	Mashed or baked potatoes
Oatmeal	Cornflakes, Cheerios
All-Bran	Watermelon
Pasta (al dente)	
Orange	

Source: Foster-Powell K, Holt SHA, and Brand-Miller, JC. "International table of glycemic index and glycemic load values: 2002." *American Journal of Clinical Nutrition* 2002; 76 (1): 5–56.

Generally speaking, in a normal diet, about 50 percent of the daily caloric intake is in the form of carbohydrates. However, in many individuals with type 2 diabetes who also have high triglycerides and low HDL cholesterol, this degree of carbohydrate intake may be too much. In these cases, it would be beneficial to reduce the overall amount of carbohydrate, yet eat foods with high fiber content.

Eating too many carbohydrates does not cause diabetes. Experiments have shown that elevated free fatty acids levels can damage beta cells. So it is possible that in a susceptible person, a high-carbohydrate diet can increase the free fatty acids to a level that can injure the islets and impair insulin secretion, but this is only a hypothesis. There is also no evidence that a high-carbohydrate diet per se (without ingestion of excess calories) leads to weight gain.

Artificial Sweeteners

Used in moderation, table sugar (sucrose) can be a part of your diet. However, if you are having problems with glucose control or you are trying to limit your carbohydrate intake (for weight loss or lowering triglycerides), reducing the amount of sugar you eat may be important to you. If this is the case, you have the option of using sweeteners that do not raise blood glucose levels. Aspartame (NutraSweet) consists of two major amino acids, aspartic acid and phenylalanine, which combine to produce a sweetener 180 times as sweet as sucrose. A major limitation is that it is not heat stable, and so it cannot be used in cooking. Saccharin (Sweet 'N Low), sucralose (Splenda), and acesulfame potassium (Sweet One) are other sweeteners that can be used in cooking and baking.

Fructose is a natural sugar substance that is a highly effective sweetener and only slightly increases blood glucose levels, and it does not require insulin for its metabolism. However, high amounts of fructose do raise triglycerides and cholesterol, so it is not really that advantageous as a sweetening agent. Of course, you can still eat fructose-containing fruits and vegetables or fructose-sweetened foods in moderation.

Sugar Alcohols

Sugar alcohols, also know as polyols or polyalcohol, are commonly used as sweeteners and bulking agents. They occur naturally in a variety of fruits and vegetables, but are also commercially made from sucrose, glucose, and starch. Examples are sorbitol, xylitol, mannitol, lactitol, isomalt, maltitol, and hydrogenated starch hydrolysates (HSH). If the food has just one sugar alcohol it will be listed separately on the food label, but if the food contains several sugar alcohols the label will just say "sugar alcohols." They are not as easily absorbed as sugar and so do not raise blood glucose levels as much. Therefore, they are often present in food products that are labeled "sugar free" such as chewing gum, lozenges, hard candy, and sugar-free ice cream. If you consume enough of these foods, however, they will raise the blood glucose, and so you need to count half the carbohydrate listed on the food label that comes from sugar alcohol. If you consume too much of these sugar alcohols, you may experience side effects such as bloating and diarrhea. If you are counting calories, remember that sugar alcohols have lower caloric content than sugar (1.5 to 3 kcals per gram as opposed to 4 kcals per gram of sugar).

FATS

Fat is necessary in moderation and important for good health. It is an important source of calories and should contribute 25 to 35 percent of daily energy requirements. Fats are necessary for the absorption of vitamins A, D, E, and K. Fat also tastes good and makes us feel full.

Understanding the fat content of a meal is important for a number of reasons. First of all, fats are the most energy-dense foods. One gram of fat contains 9 kcals, whereas a gram of proteins and carbohydrates contains 4 kcals. Therefore, fat restriction is an important part of any weight-reducing diet. Second, different kinds of fats can also affect the lipid profile and so may have an effect on development of heart disease.

Not all fats are the same—there are three types of fats:

- **Saturated fats** are found in animal fats such as lard, butter, cheese, milk, and meat and in coconut and palm kernel oil.

- **Monounsaturated fats** are found in olive oil, canola oil, and peanuts and other nuts.

- **Polyunsaturated fats** are found in vegetable oils such as safflower, corn, soybean, and sunflower oil and also in fish and seafood.

DID YOU KNOW?

What Is a Calorie?

A **calorie** is a unit of energy. A **kilocalorie** (kcal) is 1,000 calories. While it isn't scientifically correct, when people discuss food, they use the terms *calorie* and *kilocalorie* interchangeably. A food label stating that the food has 250 calories really means 250,000 calories or 250 kcals. No matter how you say it, eating more calories (or kilocalories) than your body needs results in weight gain.

A lot of foods contain a combination of these different types of fats: for example, avocados contain all three types.

Saturated fats increase LDL cholesterol, but they also increase HDL cholesterol, and so the effect of saturated fats on increasing the risk of heart disease is probably modest. What has been shown in scientific studies is that when you replace saturated fats with monounsaturated and polyunsaturated fats, you lower your total cholesterol levels and risk of heart disease. For example in the Finnish Mental Health Study, replacing a high-saturated-fat institutional diet with a polyunsaturated diet lowered the rate of heart disease by 50 to 65 percent. In the Lyon Heart Study, a diet in which fat intake came mostly from canola oil (a monounsaturated fat) was shown to decrease the likelihood of a second heart attack by 73 percent.

Trans-Fatty Acids (Trans Fats)

Trans fats are harmful because they increase the risk of heart disease. They are produced when vegetable oils are converted into semisolid fats such as margarine and vegetable shortening. They are also known as **partially hydrogenated vegetable oils**. There are some naturally produced trans fats in dairy products, but most of the trans fats in our diet are man-made. Manufacturers put them in food products to increase the product shelf life—for example, crackers stay crispy longer. The problem is that they appear to raise LDL cholesterol (the "bad" cholesterol) and lower the HDL cholesterol (the "good" cholesterol). They may also have a negative effect on the cells lining the blood vessels, promoting atherosclerosis. The FDA now requires manufacturers to list trans fats on food labels.

Omega-3 Fatty Acids

Omega-3 fatty acids are a kind of polyunsaturated fat that lowers the triglycerides and raises HDL cholesterol. There are three important omega-3 fatty acids for human nutrition:

- Alpha-linolenic acid
- Eicosapentaenoic acid
- Docosahexaenoic acid

Humans cannot synthesize omega-3 fatty acids—they must be obtained from the diet. Good dietary sources include

- Oily cold-water fish such as salmon, herring, mackerel, anchovies, and sardines
- Flaxseed oil (about 55 percent ALA), canola oil, walnut oil, soybeans, and pumpkin seeds

You may have to consume up to 3 grams of omega-3 fatty acids daily to lower your triglyceride levels. Doses higher than this may be harmful—they may increase the risk of a hemorrhagic stroke (bleeding into the brain).

Getting 1 gram of omega-3 fatty acids from fish would mean eating two or three six-ounce servings per week. There has been some concern that fish may have accumulated heavy metals such as mercury and pollutants such as PCBs and dioxin. You can get more information from the FDA/EPA (Environmental Protection Agency) dietary advice statement on mercury in fish and shellfish (see Resources).

Fortunately, you can buy a pure distilled form of omega-3 fatty acids as capsules, which can be taken as a dietary supplement. There is also a prescription product called Lovaza that your doctor can prescribe.

Cholesterol

Cholesterol is not a fat—it is a chemical that has a number of important functions:

- It is a building block for a number of important hormones, including the sex hormones testosterone and estrogen.
- It is part of the insulation around nerves.
- It is a component of the membranes surrounding all the cells in the body.
- It is the precursor for bile acids, which are important for fat absorption.

The reason that we often discuss cholesterol when talking about fats is that in the bloodstream, the particles that transport fats (as triglycerides) also transport cholesterol, and these particles (LDL, VLDL, HDL, chylomicrons) are involved in the processes that cause heart disease. A reduction in total fat consumption reduces cholesterol levels by 10 to 15 percent. The American Diabetes Association recommends that cholesterol in the diet should be less than 300 mg per day. If your LDL cholesterol level is more than 100 mg/dl, the amount of cholesterol in your diet should be less than 200 mg per day. Table 8-2 shows some foods that are high in cholesterol.

Table 8-2	Foods High in Cholesterol	
Food	**Serving Size**	**Amount of Cholesterol (mg)**
Egg yolk	1	225
Liver	3.5 oz	300
Kidney	3.5 oz	375
Butter	4 oz	248

Table 8-3 Protein Content of Some Common Foods

Food	Serving Size	Protein (g)
Medium egg	1	6
Milk	8 oz	8
Cheese	1 oz	7
Cooked chicken	3 oz	27
Peanuts	½ cup	19

PROTEINS

Protein intake for a person with diabetes should be the same as in a person who does not have diabetes. In the United States, protein accounts for about 15 to 35 percent of the total energy consumed per day, and there is no reason that people with diabetes should have a different amount. The only exception is in people with diabetic kidney disease. Too much protein can worsen the kidney disease, and so they need to restrict their protein intake to less than 0.36 grams per pound per day. For example, for a person weighing 154 pounds, 154 pounds $\times$ 0.36 = 55 grams of protein per day. Table 8-3 illustrates the protein content of some common foods.

Nutrition in Type 1 Diabetes

Most people with type 1 diabetes are of normal body weight, and they usually do not need to be on a calorie-restricted diet. They also do not tend to have the cholesterol abnormalities that are commonly seen in patients with type 2 diabetes.

The American Diabetes Association recommends that an adult should obtain

- 45 to 65 percent of the total daily kilocalories in the form of carbohydrates
- 25 to 35 percent of the total daily kilocalories in the form of fat (of which less than 7 percent are from saturated fat)
- 10 to 35 percent of the total daily kilocalories in the form of protein

These recommendations also apply to lean individuals without diabetes. In other words, this is a normal, healthy diet.

You should have a good idea of how much carbohydrate you are going to eat at a meal, because it will affect how much insulin you should take before the meal. Estimating the carbohydrate content of a meal is called **carbohydrate counting** or carbohydrate exchange. You need two pieces of information to count carbohydrates:

- You need to know the carbohydrate content of the food per unit measure.
- You need to estimate the size of the food portion (for example, by weighing it or using a measuring cup or counting slices).

You can think of food in 15-gram carbohydrate units: this is equivalent to 1 carbohydrate exchange or 1 carbohydrate unit.

There are lots of lists available (in books and on the Internet) that describe different foods, portion sizes, and carbohydrate content. Table 8-4 lists some common foods and the amount equivalent to 15 grams of carbohydrate units.

Table 8-4   Foods and Quantities Equivalent to About 15 Grams of Carbohydrate

Food	Quantity
Milk, soy milk, buttermilk	1 cup
Plain yogurt	⅔ cup
Bread	1 oz (1 slice)
Bagel (store-bought)	1 oz (¼ bagel)
Cooked rice, couscous, or pasta	⅓ cup
Hot dog bun, pita bread, English muffin	1
Cooked beans (pinto, kidney, garbanzo, lentils)	½ cup
Cooked sweet potato, potato, corn, peas, yam	½ cup
Tortilla (flour or corn)	1 (6 inch)
Popped popcorn	3 cups
Apple, banana	1 small (4 oz)
Peach, pear, nectarine, kiwi	1 (4 oz)
Pineapple chunks, blueberries, blackberries	¾ cup
Grapes	17
Orange, apple, or grapefruit juice	½ cup
Strawberries, watermelon	1¼ cups

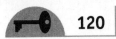

Food Labels and Fiber

The food labels on all packaged foods describe the serving size and how many grams of carbohydrates there are in each serving. One word of caution: the food labels break down the carbohydrates into sugars and fibers. Since humans cannot digest fiber very well, the grams of fiber should be excluded from the carbohydrate estimation, especially if the fiber content is particularly high. If you are going to eat a food with 5 grams of dietary fiber or more, you should subtract the dietary fiber content from the total carbohydrate. For example, for a food in which the carbohydrate content is 31 grams per serving, and there are 6 grams of dietary fiber in that serving, calculate the insulin for $31 - 6 = 25$ grams carbohydrate.

Figure 8-1 gives an example of a food label, with some comments on what you should look for when you read labels.

For each meal, count the total number of carbohydrates in all the foods (typically anywhere from 30 to 105 grams), and then inject a dose of a fast-acting insulin analog (such as lispro, aspart, or glulisine—see Chapter 6) based on the amount of carbohydrates. For example, if your insulin to carbohydrate ratio is 1 unit for 15 grams carbohydrate, for a bagel containing 60 grams carbohydrate you would give $60 \div 15 = 4$ units fast-acting insulin analog.

The insulin to carbohydrate ratio can vary according to

- The time of day
- Your age
- The duration of diabetes

Although using ratios of insulin to carbohydrate allows you to eat variable amounts of carbohydrates, some restrictions are still necessary. You should limit carbohydrates in liquid form, such as juice and regular sodas, which are rapidly absorbed. You should also bear in mind that the insulin injected can't deal very well with large amounts of carbohydrates (over 105 grams at one time). An exception to this rule is athletes, who can manage higher amounts of carbohydrates at one time (up to 150 grams).

Figure 8-1 Nutrition Facts Label

Nutrition Facts

Serving Size 1 cup (228g)
Servings Per Container 2

Amount Per Serving

Calories 250	Calories from Fat 110

	% Daily Value*
Total Fat 12g	18%
Saturated Fat 3g	15%
Trans Fat 3g	
Cholesterol 30mg	10%
Sodium 470mg	20%
Total Carbohydrate 31g	10%
Dietary Fiber 0g	0%
Sugars 5g	
Protein 5g	

Vitamin A	4%
Vitamin C	2%
Calcium	20%
Iron	4%

*Percent Daily Values are based on a 2,000 calorie diet. Your Daily Values may be higher or lower depending on your calorie needs:

	Calories:	2,000	2,500
Total Fat	Less than	65g	80g
Sat Fat	Less than	20g	25g
Cholesterol	Less than	300mg	300mg
Sodium	Less than	2,400mg	2,400mg
Total Carbohydrate		300g	375g
Dietary Fiber		25g	30g

1. Start by looking at the serving size and number of servings per container.

2. Look at calories if you are on a calorie-restricted diet.

3. Look at the other nutrients—this particular food has some trans fats, which you might want to avoid.

4. Look at the amount of carbohydrate per serving. Also pay attention to dietary fiber—if significant, then subtract the value from total carbohydrate.

Source: www.cfsan.fda.gov/~dms/foodlab.html.

WHAT ABOUT ALCOHOL?

Should you count the carbohydrates in the alcohol you drink? When you drink alcohol, it is metabolized (that is, broken down) by the liver, and there is less glucose production while the alcohol is being broken down. In people with diabetes who are on insulin, this can cause hypoglycemic reactions. It is therefore important that you drink alcohol with a meal rather than on an empty stomach. The recommended amount of alcohol is the same as for people without diabetes—two drinks for men and one for women. One drink is defined as twelve ounces of beer, five ounces of wine, or one and a half ounces of distilled spirits. You generally do not need to count the carbohydrates in the alcohol or inject any extra insulin for the alcohol. The exception would be if you drank several cans of beer at one sitting; then you may need to give some insulin for the carbohydrates in the beer.

Your Diet for Type 2 Diabetes

People with type 2 diabetes are frequently overweight, so advice about nutrition is directed not only at controlling carbohydrate intake, but also at limiting calories. (I discuss caloric restriction and weight loss in Chapter 10.) If you have type 2 diabetes, there are several reasons why you still need to estimate the carbohydrate content of your food:

- Limiting the carbohydrate intake and substituting some of the calories with monounsaturated fats can help reduce your triglyceride levels and increase HDL cholesterol levels.

- Abnormalities in insulin secretion mean that eating a high-carbohydrate meal results in high glucose levels immediately after the meal. You want to avoid these high postmeal glucose levels because they can contribute to increases in HbA1c levels (see Chapter 5).

- If you are using insulin injections, you need to count carbohydrates in order to adjust your insulin doses (just like people with type 1 diabetes).

- Estimating carbohydrate content is also important if you are taking sulfonylureas, nateglinide, or repaglinide. This is because with these medicines, too few carbohydrates can cause low glucose levels.

Summary
- According to the ADA, a normal, healthy diet for people with diabetes should consist of
  - 45 to 65 percent of total daily kilocalories from carbohydrates
  - 25 to 35 percent of total daily kilocalories from fat
  - 10 to 35 percent of total daily kilocalories from protein
- The glucose rise after eating is due to the carbohydrates in the meal, and therefore all people with diabetes should learn carbohydrate counting.
- If you are on insulin, your dose should be based on the amount of carbohydrates in your meal.
- When taken on an empty stomach, alcohol can lower glucose levels.

Salt and Potassium

High blood pressure occurs frequently in people with type 2 diabetes and with diabetic kidney disease. Reducing your salt intake can help lower the blood pressure. You can reduce the amount of salt in your diet by

- Avoiding or reducing intake of foods with high salt content such as canned foods, pickled vegetables, soy sauce, teriyaki sauce, and tomato sauce.
- Cooking with less salt. Instead, use herbs, spices, and lemon juice for flavoring.

Another element that you might need to think about in your diet is potassium. If you have diabetic kidney disease, your blood potassium levels can go up. Some medications that are used to treat high blood pressure (for example, the ACE inhibitors) can also raise your blood potassium levels. This is of concern because very high levels of potassium can affect the heart rhythm. So if you have high potassium levels, you will need to limit or avoid foods that are high in potassium, for example bananas and tomatoes.

- Dietary recommendations include:
  - Restrict calories if overweight or obese.
  - Reduce cholesterol and trans fats to reduce risk of heart disease.
  - Limit carbohydrates to avoid very high glucose levels after meals. Eat foods that have a high fiber content and a low glycemic index and have not been highly processed.
  - Replace carbohydrates with monounsaturated and polyunsaturated fats to lower triglycerides and raise HDL cholesterol levels.
  - Take omega-3 fatty acids with medical supervision to lower triglyceride levels.

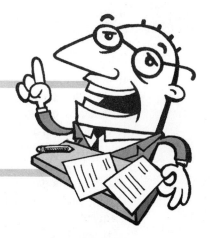

CHAPTER 9

Developing a Safe Exercise Program

A regular exercise program has many benefits for everyone. These include:

- An improved sense of well-being
- Stress reduction
- Lower blood pressure
- Lower cholesterol and increased HDL cholesterol
- Improved muscle tone and reduced risk of falls
- Better sleep
- Weight loss and maintenance
- Maintenance of bone strength
- Less risk of heart disease

If you have diabetes, you will get all these benefits from exercise. In addition, regular exercise will improve your insulin sensitivity, and if you have type 2 diabetes, regular exercise will also improve your glucose control. However, there are a number of challenges to exercising safely if you have diabetes. The challenges

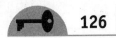

include avoiding both high and low blood glucose levels during exercise, especially when you are on insulin, and how to exercise safely when you have complications of diabetes, especially neuropathy and heart disease.

Exercise has numerous benefits for people with diabetes, but it is not as simple as saying "go and exercise." Before embarking on an exercise plan, visit your physician and diabetes educator and get guidance on how to exercise safely. If you have type 1 diabetes, you may need to adjust your insulin and your carbohydrate intake before, during, and after exercise. You will also need to monitor your glucose levels more frequently.

If you have type 2 diabetes, you may also need to cut back on the insulin or oral medicines that can cause hypoglycemia. Additional modifications of the exercise plan may be necessary if you have complications of diabetes.

Acute Versus Chronic Exercise

You can think of exercise in two ways:

- Acute exercise, which means one bout of exercise
- Chronic exercise, which means regular, frequent exercise, also known as exercise training

Acute and chronic exercise have different effects on the body. One important difference that is relevant to diabetes is the effect on insulin sensitivity. A single bout of exercise will increase your insulin sensitivity, but this effect is rapidly lost within twenty-four hours. On the other hand, chronic exercise (exercise training) leads to an increase in insulin sensitivity that can last up to two weeks after stopping exercise. If you are taking insulin for glucose control and you do not reduce the dose when your body becomes more insulin sensitive, you will have low glucose reactions. If, however, you stop exercising regularly, your improved insulin sensitivity will wear off, and your glucose levels will go up unless you increase your insulin.

The impact of exercise on insulin sensitivity depends on the intensity of your exercise as well as the total amount of exercise you do per week. It appears that the amount of exercise has a bigger effect than the intensity—in other words, more total minutes of moderate exercise a week has a greater effect on insulin sensitivity than more intense exercise for fewer times per week.

Although this chapter is principally about planned exercise activity, the information also applies to unplanned exercise such as running for the bus or climbing stairs. Other heavy physical work such as gardening, cleaning house, and moving furniture can also be considered as acute bouts of exercise.

Types of Exercise

We'll discuss four types of exercise: aerobic, resistance training, flexibility, and anaerobic.

AEROBIC EXERCISE (CARDIORESPIRATORY ENDURANCE)

During aerobic exercise, there is sustained physical activity. The heart rate and breathing rate increase to supply additional oxygen and fuel to the muscles. Walking, bicycling, jogging, swimming, and racquet sports are examples of aerobic exercise.

The American College of Sports Medicine defines moderate exercise as 55 to 69 percent of maximal heart rate; hard (or higher intensity) exercise as 70 to 89 percent of maximal heart rate; and very hard exercise as 90 percent of the maximal heart rate and above. You can determine whether your exercise is moderate or intense in several ways:

- **Measure your heart rate using a heart rate monitor.** Your maximal heart rate will vary depending on your age and gender. A simple formula is to subtract your age from 220 for men and from 226 for women. There are also a number of websites that will calculate your heart rate for different levels of exercise and your age and gender. You can also go on a treadmill with a pulse monitor and run an intense program supervised by a fitness coach to determine your maximal heart rate.

- **The talk test.** This is a simple way of determining if your exercise level is too high. If it is just possible to hold a conversation while you are exercising, then your exercise level is moderate. However, if you are having a hard time getting your words out, then the exercise intensity is greater than the recommended range (that is, it is vigorous exercise).

- **Assessing your perception.** Evaluate how hard are you exercising by your breathing rate and level of fatigue. In the Borg perceived exertion scale (see Figure 9-1), you would rank this on a scale of 6 to 20, where 6 is no exertion and 20 is maximal exertion.

So, if you feel that your exercise is at a scale of 9 (very light), you should increase it. But if you feel the exercise is at a scale of 19 (extremely hard), you should back off. Scales of 12 to 14 (somewhat hard) are considered moderate exercise. You can multiply the number for the perceived exertion by 10 to give you an approximate heart rate. For example, if you think you are exercising at a scale of 12, your heart rate is in the range of $12 \times 10 = 120$ beats per minute.

Figure 9-1   Borg Rate of Perceived Exertion

6	7	8	9	10	11	12	13	14	15	16	17	18	19	20
No exertion			Very light exertion		Light exertion		Somewhat hard		Hard		Very hard		Extremely hard	

Source: Borg, G. *Borg's Perceived Exertion and Pain Scales.* Stockholm: Human Kinetics, 1998.

This method of assessing intensity of exercise is favored if you have autonomic neuropathy or if you are taking medications such as beta-blockers, when measuring the heart rate to determine exercise intensity is not accurate.

The U.S. surgeon general recommends that most people should have a moderate level of aerobic exercise for thirty minutes or more five times a week. Types of moderate aerobic exercise include a brisk walk, bicycling (at a speed less than 10 mph), and doubles tennis. Vigorous aerobic exercise is jogging, swimming, bicycling (at a speed greater than 10 mph), and competitive sports such as basketball and squash. For weight maintenance, sixty minutes of moderate exercise five days per week may be necessary.

RESISTANCE EXERCISE (STRENGTH TRAINING)

Resistance exercise is using your muscle strength to move a weight—for example, weight lifting and weight machines. It increases muscle strength and, like aerobic exercise, improves insulin sensitivity.

Resistance or strength training using exercise machines involving multiple exercises (three sets three times a week) has been shown to significantly improve glucose control and appears to be safe. Each weight should weigh just enough so that you can't lift it more than eight to ten times a set. Blood glucose monitoring is necessary for this type of exercise.

FLEXIBILITY EXERCISE (STRETCHING)

This type of exercise helps to maintain or increase the range of motion at joints. Yoga and tai chi are examples of such exercises.

There is no good scientific evidence that stretching reduces muscle injury, but most people tend to feel good when they stretch at the beginning and at the end of their exercise session. Although stretching usually does not have a significant effect on glucose control, in some people with type 1 diabetes, just the relaxation that comes from stretching can cause a fall in glucose levels. It is a good idea to check a few times to make sure that this is not happening to you.

ANAEROBIC EXERCISE

Anaerobic exercise is brief and intense exercise in which oxygen is not necessary for producing the energy needed by the exercising muscles. Sprinting, power lifting, and jumping are examples of anaerobic exercises.

Exercise and Type 1 Diabetes

If you have type 1 diabetes, and you are not in the honeymoon period when the beta cells still have some capacity to make insulin, you can have fluctuating blood glucose levels, and exercise can be particularly tricky. You may encounter the following problems while exercising:

DID YOU KNOW?

Regulating Glucose Levels During Exercise

The delivery and use of different fuels by the body at rest and during exercise depends on the action of the sympathetic nervous system and actions of insulin and glucagon. Having an understanding of these actions will help explain why exercise in diabetes can cause both high and low glucose levels and even lead to diabetic ketoacidosis (DKA):

- At rest, muscles mostly use fatty acids as their energy source. When you exercise, this changes. With short, intense exercise, the muscles switch to using glucose. The sympathetic nervous system facilitates this switch in fuel use. It turns off insulin release and stimulates fat cells to release glycerol and fatty acids. The fall in insulin allows the liver to make and release more glucose.

- The liver has an ability to release a lot of glucose, and when exercise is intense, glucose levels actually go up immediately after exercise. Usually the insulin goes up as well (two- to threefold) to regulate this postexercise glucose rise.

- After exercise, the glucose uptake by the muscle continues—this replenishes the glycogen stores of the muscles and the liver.

- Delivery of insulin into the body by subcutaneous (just-under-the-skin) injection makes it difficult to reduce the insulin levels at the start of exercise—this is particularly true in the case of unexpected exercise. The high insulin levels prevent the liver from making sufficient glucose to maintain normal blood glucose levels, and you can become hypoglycemic during exercise.

- With intense exercise, the increased activity of the sympathetic nervous system can make the glucose go up during and especially after exercise. The rise after exercise can be problematic if the insulin levels remain low.

- If you participate in a competitive sport, the stress of competition and the adrenaline rush can lead to insulin resistance and increased glucose levels before exercise.

- Many hours after exercise, the muscles and the liver continue to take up glucose from the blood in order to replenish their glycogen stores. So, in order to avoid hypoglycemia some hours after exercise, you need to decrease your insulin dose or increase your carbohydrate intake.

- With regular exercise (the training effect), your insulin requirements will generally fall. You will be more insulin sensitive, so you will need to adjust your basal and bolus insulin doses.

- Exercise can accelerate insulin absorption, especially if the site of injection is near the exercising muscle (for example, the thigh).

If your blood insulin levels are low and your glucose level is high before exercise, the combination of high glucose production by the liver and free fatty acid production from the fat stores during exercise can result in high glucose levels and production of ketones, which can lead to DKA. Therefore you have to be cautious about exercising if your glucose is above 250 to 300 mg/dl, especially if you also have urinary ketones.

RECOMMENDATIONS FOR EXERCISE IN TYPE 1 DIABETES

If you have type 1 diabetes, consider taking the following steps.

Keep an Exercise Log

Write down when you are exercising, the relation to the previous meal and insulin bolus, the type of exercise, the duration and intensity, how much carbohydrate (CHO) was consumed before, during, and after exercise, and blood glucose levels (see Figure 9-2). This information is essential for making appropriate changes the next time you exercise.

Figure 9-2   Example of an Exercise Log

Date		Before			During			After		
Activity	Time									
	CHO									
	Bolus									
	Basal									
Comments										

Plan Your Exercise

Plan how long you will exercise, how intense it will be, and how soon after a meal you will exercise. Try to be consistent from day to day.

Monitor Blood Glucose Levels

Take your glucose meter with you when you exercise, and check your blood glucose levels before, during (at least once or twice), and after exercise. If possible check them at least two or three times at half-hour intervals before the exercise to find out the direction of glucose changes. Prick your finger for the blood sample—do not use your forearm, because there may be a five- to twenty-minute lag in the glucose response in the arm.

With intense exercise, be prepared for lower glucose levels several hours after exercise, for example, in the middle of the night. Have a bedtime snack, or wake up and check your blood glucose.

Adjust the Insulin Dose

Before exercise, adjust the bolus or basal insulin, or both, in anticipation of the exercise.

- A bolus of a fast-acting insulin analog lasts for about four hours, and the peak is at about one to one and a half hours. If you exercise within two hours, you will need to cut back on the premeal bolus (to 50 to 75 percent of your usual dose).

- Making an adjustment in basal insulin dosing is easier if you are on an insulin pump. If you are planning for exercise of long duration (longer than ninety minutes), you may want to cut back the amount of your basal insulin for up to two hours before the exercise. If you are participating in competitive sports, you may find that the "adrenaline rush" means that you may have to increase your basal insulin temporarily for up to two hours before the exercise.

- Adjusting the basal dosage of the long-acting insulins like glargine or detemir is trickier—you can try cutting back to 50 to 80 percent of the dose on the days you exercise. Any high glucose levels earlier in the day can be covered by giving additional bolus insulin.

During exercise your options will depend whether you are on a pump or on injections.

- If you are on the pump, you have a number of options as to what to do regarding the basal insulin delivery. For short-duration exercise lasting an hour or so, you can simply come off the pump. If the pump is taken off for more than an hour (for example, while swimming), a small bolus may be given before coming off. If you will be exercising for several hours, a temporary basal amount (20 to 75 percent of your usual dose) might be necessary. For example, if you go cross-country skiing for several hours, you may change your basal to 20 to 50 percent of your usual dose for the duration of the exercise. A similar change may be required for a marathon.

- If you are on insulin glargine or detemir, you do not have the option of changing the basal rate during exercise: your only option is to consume additional carbohydrates.

After exercise you will adjust the bolus and basal insulins for the acute effects of exercise and also for the effects of chronic exercise.

- If you get predictably high glucose levels after exercise, be prepared to give a little bolus of a fast-acting insulin analog. With intense and/ or prolonged exercise, hypoglycemia can occur several hours (up to twelve to sixteen hours) afterward, and you should be prepared to reduce the basal insulin (or eat a snack). You might consider purchasing a continuous glucose monitoring system that can alert you to overnight hypoglycemia.

- After a weekend of increased physical activity such as skiing, a reduction in insulin requirements may persist for an additional twenty-four hours.

- With exercise training, you may become more insulin sensitive, and you may need to change your usual insulin regimen by cutting back on both basal and bolus insulin doses.

Eat Carbohydrates

For athletes with diabetes, it is recommended that 55 to 60 percent of the total daily kilocalories should be carbohydrates. Endurance athletes (such as long-distance runners or cyclists) should consider eating a carbohydrate-rich meal (1 to 2 grams of carbohydrate per kilogram of body weight) about three to four hours before exercising to maximize pre-exercise glycogen stores. If the exercise is unplanned, eat 20 to 30 grams of carbohydrate immediately before you exercise.

The amount of carbohydrate that needs to be consumed will depend on the duration and intensity of the exercise. Generally speaking, about 20 to 30 grams of carbohydrate is needed for each thirty minutes of exercise. Table 9-1 provides a good starting point in determining how many grams of carbohydrate you might need every half hour for different types of exercise.

The type of carbohydrate you consume can vary:

- Before exercise, you could have fruit (apples, dried apricots), bread, yogurt, porridge, pasta, or milk.

- During exercise, you could have a fruit juice/water mixture or sports drink. Sports drinks can give you some sodium and potassium as well as carbohydrate. Read the labels for the carbohydrate, sodium, and potassium

Table 9-1 Approximate Amounts of Carbohydrate for Different Levels of Exercise	
Type of Exercise	**Approximate Grams Carbohydrate per 30 Minutes of Exercise for a 150-Pound Person**
Leisurely walk	10
Tennis (doubles), golf, bicycling (6 mph), painting, raking leaves	15
Vigorous dancing, brisk walking	20
Moderate basketball, bicycling (10 mph), shoveling snow, swimming (slow crawl)	25
Soccer, digging, running (5 mph), waterskiing	30
Cross-country skiing (5 mph), vigorous ice skating, bicycle racing, mountain climbing, swimming (fast crawl)	50
Source: Adapted from Walsh J, Roberts R. *Pumping Insulin*, 3rd ed. San Diego, CA: Torrey Pines Press, 2000.	

contents. Sport gels or carbohydrate-rich bars are also good sources of rapidly absorbed carbohydrates and salts—usually, you want to drink some water with them.

- After exercise, you can have bread, potato, rice, cereal such as cornflakes, a granola bar, or cookies.

Drink Fluids

Dehydration will increase your glucose levels, so you need to drink plenty of fluids while exercising. In the two hours before exercise, drink two glasses of water, and during exercise, drink enough to replace fluid loss. For prolonged exercise such as running or cycling, drinking approximately 250 ml (8 ounces) every twenty minutes of exercise would be reasonable. Sport drinks are good for fluid and carbohydrate replacement. Avoid drinking too much fluid, because this can lead to low sodium levels.

Provide Emergency Information

Wear your MedicAlert bracelet or shoe tags, just in case you get a severe episode of hypoglycemia.

Exercise and Type 2 Diabetes

If you have type 2 diabetes and you are on insulin, you will face issues similar to those of a person with type 1 diabetes (see the tips and advice in the preceding section), except that generally, your glucose levels will be more stable. This is principally because most patients with type 2 diabetes still have functioning beta cells in their pancreas, with a significant contribution of their own insulin.

If you take oral diabetes medications, you cannot assume that your health will be fine when you exercise: if you take sulfonylureas, nateglinide, or repaglinide, you can get low glucose levels with exercise. Prepare for this by taking your meter and some glucose tablets or juice with you. If hypoglycemia occurs when you exercise, talk to your doctor about reducing the dose of your sulfonylurea medication.

EXERCISE IN THE PRESENCE OF DIABETES COMPLICATIONS

If you have any complications of diabetes, you need to take them into account when you are planning your exercise.

Nervous System Complications

Nerve damage to the feet can stop you from recognizing injury, and as a result you can develop calluses, foot ulcers, or even a Charcot's foot (see Chapter 3). If you have significant peripheral neuropathy, you should avoid pounding the pavement and try non-weight-bearing exercises such as swimming, rowing, and cycling instead. When you buy athletic footwear, choose shoes with cushioned midsoles and socks that wick away moisture.

Autonomic neuropathy can dull the classic warning signs of hypoglycemia (**palpitations**, sweating, and shaking), and this may prevent you from recognizing exercise-induced hypoglycemia. Similarly, if you have hypoglycemic unawareness due to recurrent hypoglycemic episodes, you should monitor your blood glucose more frequently during and after exercise.

Autonomic neuropathy can also cause problems with blood pressure regulation, and you can get light-headed with exercise. Dehydration can worsen the problem, so it is important to drink adequate fluids. The heart rate is often increased even at rest, and this means that you cannot rely on taking your pulse rate to monitor your exercise level. It may be best to judge the intensity of your exercise on your perception: if you think the exercise is somewhat hard, this is equivalent to moderate exercise (see the Borg perceived exertion scale in the "Aerobic Exercise" section earlier in this chapter).

Diabetic Eye Disease

If you have retinopathy, vigorous exercise, weight lifting, or boxing may precipitate bleeding, and therefore you should see your ophthalmologist before embarking on a vigorous exercise program.

Heart Disease

Type 2 diabetes increases the risk of coronary artery disease, and therefore you should get an evaluation for heart disease prior to starting an exercise program. Older people with type 2 diabetes who are just planning moderate activity such as walking may not need any special evaluation. However, if you were previously inactive and are planning a vigorous exercise program, or you have autonomic neuropathy or previous heart problems, you should get a cardiac stress test. Your doctor may do a test called thallium-201 scintigraphy, which looks for areas of the heart that have insufficient blood flow. You can estimate your risk for heart disease using the ADA Diabetes Personal Health Decisions online questionnaire (see Resources).

Summary

- Exercise has many benefits for people with diabetes. Before embarking on an exercise plan, visit your physician and diabetes educator for guidance on how to exercise safely.

- In type 1 diabetes, you may need to adjust your insulin and carbohydrate intake before, during, and after exercise. You will also need to monitor your glucose levels more frequently.

  - During exercise, you usually need less insulin. If you are on a pump you can cut back on the basal insulin. If you are on injections you may need to take additional carbohydrate.

  - Several hours after intense or prolonged exercise, your glucose level can go low, so check your glucose and cut back on the basal insulin or eat a snack.

  - With exercise training, you will become more insulin sensitive, and you will need less basal and bolus insulin.

- In type 2 diabetes, you may need to cut back on the insulin or oral medicines that can cause hypoglycemia when you exercise.

- If you have complications of diabetes, additional modifications of the exercise plan may be necessary:

  - If you have severe peripheral neuropathy and foot deformity, non-weight-bearing exercises like swimming and cycling are safer.

  - Avoid vigorous exercise, weight lifting, or boxing if you have active retinal bleeding.

- If you are normally sedentary and plan to start a vigorous exercise program, you may need to get a cardiac stress test.

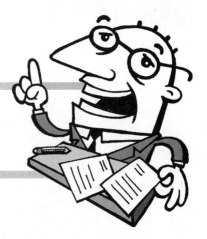

CHAPTER 10

Weight Loss

Being overweight or obese (especially when the fat is in the abdomen) increases the body's insulin needs, and losing this extra weight can significantly improve diabetes control. Often the weight loss can eliminate the need for medications altogether. You do not have to lose a huge amount of weight—a 5 percent loss in body weight is sufficient.

Basic Weight-Loss Concepts

There are many approaches to weight loss, and I will discuss these briefly. First, here are some basic concepts about weight loss:

- **Weight loss occurs when there is a negative energy balance.** If you consume fewer kilocalories than you expend, you will lose weight. This is the principle behind all weight-loss diets, and there are no exceptions to this rule. If you reduce the number of calories you eat by about 500 kilocalories per day, you will lose about one pound in weight per week.

- **Physiologically, we are designed to avoid eating too little.** The mechanisms of the body evolved when there was less food available than we have now, and these mechanisms are designed to avoid weight loss. With environmental changes and the ready availability of highly dense calories (that is, lots of calories in a small portion size), it takes very little excess caloric intake on a daily basis to gain a considerable amount of weight over time. It is estimated that in the United States, over 90 percent of the weight gain seen in adults results from a positive energy balance of *less than 100 kcal a day*. It is very easy to get into a positive energy balance (more calories consumed than expended)—for example, a two-ounce candy bar such as Snickers has 273 kcals.

• **The body's energy requirement goes down when you lose weight and as you age.** About 70 percent of your energy requirement is for the basic life processes, and the other 30 percent is for activity related to eating, working, and walking. Your energy requirements go down as you age and as your weight goes down. So as you lose weight, your energy requirements fall, and you will need to reduce the number of calories you consume further for continued weight loss.

Ideal Body Weight and Body Mass Index

There are relatively simple formulas that you can use to calculate your ideal body weight (IBW), your body mass index (BMI), and the number of calories you should eat each day.

IDEAL BODY WEIGHT

To determine your ideal body weight, use the following formula:

- **Men:** 106 pounds for the first 5 feet and add 6 pounds for every additional inch over 5 feet.
- **Women:** 100 pounds for the first 5 feet and add 5 pounds for every additional inch over 5 feet.

If you are large-framed you can add 10 percent to the calculated weight. For example, if you are a male who is 5 feet 8 inches tall, your ideal body weight is 106 + 48 = 154 pounds. If you are large-framed, you might weigh as much as 169 pounds.

THE BODY MASS INDEX (BMI)

BMI is a measure to estimate the degree of obesity. High BMIs are associated with increased health risks such as diabetes, heart disease, and death. To calculate your BMI, you will need your weight and height measurements. Your BMI equals your weight in pounds times 703 divided by your height in inches squared. So, for a woman

Table 10-1   Weight Classification by BMI

Weight Classification	BMI
Underweight	< 18.5
Normal	18.5 to 24.9
Overweight	25 to 29.9
Obese class I	30 to 34.9
Obese class II	35 to 39.9
Obese class III (extreme obesity)	> 40

who is 5 feet 3 inches tall (63 inches) and weighs 145 pounds, the BMI will be: 145 × 703 = 101,935, and divide that by 63 squared (3,969): 101,935 ÷ 3,969 = 25.7.

Table 10-1 summarizes how the National Institutes of Health (NIH) classifies obesity using BMI ranges. It is important to remember that body shape is also important—fat at the waist being worse than fat at the hips. Also, some people, like bodybuilders, who may have a large muscle mass and low fat, can have the same BMI as someone else who has more body fat.

Daily Energy Requirements

The amount of energy (that is, the number of calories) that you need to consume depends on your age, gender, body size, and activity level. You can calculate your daily energy requirements by calculating your **resting energy expenditure (REE)**— that is, the energy expended at rest without exposure to cold—and then multiplying this figure by an activity factor based on physical activity. Table 10-2 gives some examples.

There are lots of energy calculators available online. A relatively simple calculation for the REE is:*

Men: REE = 10 × weight (kg) + 6.25 × height (cm) − 5 × age (in years) + 5

Women: REE = 10 × weight (kg) + 6.25 × height (cm) − 5 × age (in years) − 161

Note: 1 kilogram = 2.2 pounds; 1 inch = 2.54 centimeters

---

*From Miffin MD, St Jeor ST, Hill LA, Scott BJ, Daugherty SA, Koh YO. "A new predictive equation for resting energy expenditure in healthy individuals." *Am J Clin Nutr* 1990; 51:241–47.

Table 10-2 Activity Factors Based on Physical Activity		
	Male	**Female**
Light (office work, walking, laundry, golf, restaurant work)	1.6	1.5
Moderate (light manual labor, cycling, tennis, dancing, weeding, hoeing)	1.7	1.6
Heavy (agricultural labor, athletics, mining, steel working, walking uphill with a load)	2.1	1.9

Source: Adapted from http://cals.arizona.edu/pubs/health/az1390.pdf.

For example, take a 50-year-old man who weighs 154 pounds and is 5 feet 7 inches tall. This is the same as 70 kg (154 ÷ 2.2) and 170 cm (67 inches × 2.54). This person will have an REE of 700 + 1,062.5 − 250 + 5 = 1,517. If he works in an office, his daily energy requirements are 2,427 kcals (1,517 × 1.6). If he is a gardener, the value is 2,579 kcals, and if he is agricultural laborer it is 3,186 kcals.

For obese individuals (that is, those who are greater than 125 percent of their ideal body weight), the REE calculation requires you to use an adjusted body weight value. The formula for this is: IBW + ¼ (actual weight − IBW). Thus, if your ideal body weight was 154 pounds (70 kg) and you weighed 198 pounds (90 kg), your adjusted body weight for the REE calculation is 70 + ¼ (90 − 70) = 75 kg or 165 pounds.

Weight-Loss Diets

All weight-loss diets are based on the principle of decreased caloric intake and varying amount of proteins, fats, and carbohydrates (the macronutrients). The differences between the diets are principally regarding the ratios of macronutrients and, to a lesser degree, the sources of the macronutrients—such as vegetable or animal protein or saturated or polyunsaturated fats:

> • **Balanced diets:** In these diets, the emphasis is not on severely limiting one particular macronutrient, but on eating a balanced diet with decreased caloric intake. The diet recommended by the ADA falls into this category. WeightWatchers, Jenny Craig, and eDiets are also balanced diets with an

emphasis on calorie counting. Jenny Craig and eDiets use prepared meals to control the caloric intake per meal.

• **High-protein diets:** These diets emphasize high protein intake and severely restricting carbohydrates (5 to 10 percent). Examples of high-protein diets are

  • The **Atkins Diet** (no restrictions on protein and fat sources)
  • The **South Beach Diet** (emphasizes low-glycemic carbohydrates and preferences for monounsaturated and polyunsaturated fats)

There are some diets where high protein is recommended, but not to the same extent as in the Atkins or South Beach diets, and there is more carbohydrate intake. Examples of these diets are

  • The **Zone Diet** (in which every meal needs to be 30 percent protein, 30 percent fat, and 40 percent carbohydrates)
  • The **CSIRO (Commonwealth Scientific and Industrial Research Organization) Total Wellbeing Diet** (Australian)

• **Fat-restricted diets:** These diets stress eating less energy-dense foods, such as carbohydrates and proteins (a gram of fat contains 9 kcal, compared to 4 kcal in a gram of protein or carbohydrate). Very low fat diets, in which fats are less than 10 percent of energy intake, include

  • The **Pritikin Diet** (nonvegetarian)
  • The **Ornish Diet** (vegetarian—you can eat eggs and dairy products)
  • The **McDougall Diet** (vegetarian)

THE BEST APPROACH: A LOW-CALORIE BALANCED DIET, BEHAVIOR MODIFICATION, AND INCREASED PHYSICAL ACTIVITY

Studies show that the best weight-loss and weight-maintenance results are obtained by structured programs that emphasize a combination of three interventions:

• A low-calorie balanced diet
• Behavior modification
• Increased physical activity

The ADA recommends this type of structured program for people with diabetes. So you can try the following approach to losing weight:

Reduce Calories

Your nutritionist can help you determine your energy needs, educate you about the caloric content of foods, and help you devise a diet that will allow you to be in a negative energy balance. First, limit fat intake to less than 30 percent of calories because fat is the most energy-dense nutrient. Second, control your portion size. A key approach to weight control is to eat foods that you enjoy in moderation. The plate method is helpful in controlling portions and meal composition. Take a nine-inch plate and fill a quarter of it with lean protein such as lean meat the size of your palm; another quarter with starch such as bread, rice, pasta, or starchy vegetables; and half the plate with leafy vegetables, carrots, or broccoli. The food should not be piled up (no more than one inch thick). You can also have one serving of fruit (a small apple or orange) and one serving of dairy (one cup of milk or a small dish of sugar-free pudding). For breakfast, use half the plate (one-quarter for meat and one-quarter for starch) and leave the other half empty, and for lunch and dinner use the whole plate. This gives you about 1,400 kcals daily.

Change Behavior

Eating patterns and activity are learned behaviors, and so they can be modified. In a behavior modification program, you do the following:

- **Set specific goals.** Plan a regular meal pattern, always sit down when you eat, and lengthen meal duration by ten minutes. Use low-fat, low-calorie foods and set specific goals, such as losing one pound a week. Introduce regular physical activity into your day (see next section).

- **Self-monitor.** Keep a detailed record of the foods you eat so that you do not underestimate your daily caloric intake. Be a fat detective—read food labels and think about the fat content of food that you eat. It is very easy to underestimate caloric intake. Monitor physical activity—get a pedometer and use it to monitor the amount of walking you do.

- **Control triggers.** Identify the things that promote negative eating behaviors. Keep only healthy snacks at home, and avoid vending machines at work. Also, watching television is a major barrier to physical activity.

- **Solve problems.** Once you have set a goal, try to identify factors that facilitate or hinder the goal. For example, if eating while watching television causes excess caloric intake, try eating in the kitchen or dining room without the TV. If you cannot achieve the goal, identify new approaches to overcome the barriers. Successful weight management is based on skills that can be learned and practiced.

• **Change the way you think.** Your thoughts (cognitions) directly affect your feelings and behaviors. Having negative thoughts can lead to negative behavior. For example, if you overeat and then feel like a failure, you may go on to eat even more. Identify negative thought patterns and learn to counter them with positive statements. If needed, a cognitive therapist can help you set realistic goals for weight and behavior change. Make small changes rather than large ones—they give you successful experiences to build on.

Increase Exercise/Physical Activity

Physical activity alone is not very effective in causing weight loss: you may lose only 2 to 3 percent of your excess weight. Physical activity will, however, let you keep off the weight that you lose with a reduced-calorie diet. So introduce physical activity into your day, such as taking stairs instead of elevators, walking up escalators, and parking the car farther away from your destination so you walk more. Participate in moderate physical activity (defined as burning more than 300 kcals per hour) such as walking, bicycling, or tennis for sixty minutes five times a week for long-term weight maintenance (see Chapter 9).

In a research study called the Diabetes Prevention Program, individuals with a combination of physical activity of at least 150 minutes per week, a low-calorie, low-fat diet, and behavioral approaches were able to maintain a 5 to 7 percent weight loss for an average of 2.8 years. When the National Weight Control Registry followed five thousand individuals who were able to maintain an average weight loss of sixty-six pounds for six years, they found that these individuals initially used a combination of diet and physical activity to lose the weight. Continuing the low-fat diet, monitoring food intake and calories, and moderate physical activity (sixty minutes per day) allowed these individuals to keep the weight off.

OTHER DIETS: DO THEY WORK, AND ARE THERE BENEFITS OF ONE OVER THE OTHER?

This question has received a lot of attention because of the popularity of the high-protein diets and claims by their proponents that restricting carbohydrates and allowing an unlimited intake of proteins and fats leads to significant weight loss.

Low-Carbohydrate Diets

Several studies have compared the Atkins type of low-carbohydrate diet with a low-fat diet, and these studies have found that at six months, people on the low-carbohydrate, high-protein diet had indeed lost more weight than the people on the low-fat diets, but by twelve months both groups had lost the same amount of weight. A significant proportion of subjects in both groups dropped out of the study by one year (up to 50 percent in some studies). Since the studies were for one year only, it is hard to determine if one diet or the other would be detrimental to health. What was noted was that those on the Atkins diet had lower triglycerides and higher HDL cholesterol, whereas those on the low-fat diet had lower LDL cholesterol levels. There are no studies, however, that look at long-term benefits or hazards of the low-carbohydrate, high-protein diets, and so the ADA does not recommend them.

If you have evidence of diabetic kidney disease, do not do the Atkins or South Beach diets because the high protein intake may worsen the injury to the kidneys. A diet very high in animal protein (especially red meat) and low in fiber over a long period of time may also increase the risk of gastrointestinal problems, including colon cancer.

Why does the Atkins diet cause weight loss in the short term? It is not because a high-protein diet leads to increased energy expenditure. It is possible that the high-protein diet is more satiating, and therefore you eat less. The diet is also rather monotonous, and so you may eat less. This probably also explains why patients do not continue on the diet for the long term.

Low-Fat Diets

Low-fat diets do cause weight loss, and the Ornish diet has been shown to be beneficial in reducing heart disease. However, in the long term, they have not been shown to be better than conventional diets.

Very Low Calorie Diets

These diets are recommended for people with a BMI greater than 30. The daily caloric intake is less than 800 kcals, given in the form of liquid meals. Typically, the diet consists of 70 to 100 grams protein, 80 grams carbohydrate, and 15 grams fat, plus 100 percent of recommended daily vitamins and minerals. The weight loss is usually 3.3 to 5.5 pounds per week. Generally, people enrolling in these diets lose up to 25 percent of their initial weight in the first three to four months. After the rapid weight loss over a three-month period, regular food is reintroduced and weight stabilized over the next three to four months. Unfortunately, a significant number of individuals then regain the lost weight over the next one to two years, and over the long term, these diets do not appear to be any better than low-calorie diets with conventional food. About 25 to 50 percent of people drop out of these programs within three to six months. Gallstones have been shown to develop with very low calorie diets—they may occur in as many as 25 percent of patients, and about 6 percent require surgery. The risk of gallstones is reduced if you increase the fat content of the diet, limit weight loss to 3.3 pounds per week, and give capsules of a bile salt called ursodeoxycholic acid. Other side effects of these diets include hair loss, headache, fatigue, dizziness, dehydration, muscle cramps, and constipation. If you do go on a very low calorie diet, a doctor will check you every two weeks or so while you are losing a lot of weight.

Low-Calorie Diets with Partial Meal Replacement with Liquid Meals

These are conventional low-calorie diets (1,000 to 1,500 kcals), but instead of regular food, one or more meals are replaced by liquid meals (Optifast or Slim-Fast). In one study, patients were able to lose 10 percent of their excess weight and keep it off for five years using one or two meal replacements with liquid food per day. One reason these liquid meal replacements work is because it takes the guesswork out of estimating calories. It is clearly harder to estimate portions and caloric content of conventional foods, and it has been shown that obese individuals tend to underestimate their caloric intake by 40 to 50 percent when consuming conventional foods.

Drugs for Weight Loss

There are three medications approved by the FDA for weight loss:

- Phentermine (suppresses appetite)
- Sibutramine (suppresses appetite)
- Orlistat (causes a malabsorption of fats)
- Rimonabant (suppresses appetite; not available in the United States)

In general, medications for weight loss are only modestly effective, and their main use is in conjunction with diet and exercise weight-loss interventions. The current experience suggests that the weight is regained once the drugs are stopped; in other words, the medications do not change the body, and continued use may be necessary for maintenance of weight loss.

PHENTERMINE (ADIPEX-P, ANOXINE-AM, FASTIN, IONAMIN, OBEPHEN, OBERMINE, OBESTIN-30, PHENTROL, TERAMINE)

Phentermine works on the brain—it is chemically related to amphetamine, and it helps weight loss by reducing appetite and increasing metabolism. It increases heart rate and blood pressure because it stimulates the sympathetic system. Therefore, it should not be used by people who have heart disease or high blood pressure or an overactive thyroid. Its other side effects include dry mouth, anxiety, and constipation. It has been approved for weight-loss use for up to a maximum of three months, in conjunction with diet and exercise, in people with a BMI of 27 or more who also have diabetes. The dose is 8 mg half an hour before each meal, three times a day. There are also long-acting forms given as a single dose in the morning (15 to 37.5 mg).

Despite the fact that the medication has been available for almost fifty years, long- term safety studies are lacking. The longest study was for six months, and the average weight-loss effect in combination with lifestyle changes was about eight pounds.

SIBUTRAMINE (MERIDIA)

This medication works in the brain to reduce appetite by its effect on nerve terminals that release serotonin and noradrenaline. Its side effects include insomnia, dry mouth, and increased heart rate and blood pressure. The usual starting dose is 10 mg once a day, increased to 15 mg at four weeks if the weight loss is less than four pounds. In a two-year study, people taking sibutramine were better able to keep off their weight than those taking placebo (43 percent versus 16 percent). There is no information regarding safety and benefits beyond two years.

ORLISTAT (XENICAL, TETRAHYDROLIPOSTATIN)

Orlistat blocks the activity of a pancreatic enzyme called lipase, which breaks down many fats so they can be absorbed. A 120 mg capsule is given three times a day with each main meal, and it blocks the absorption of 30 percent of ingested fat. It can cause oily stool and occasionally fecal incontinence and increased stool frequency. These unpleasant effects are the main reason why patients stop the medication—in a large two-year clinical trial about a quarter of the subjects dropped out within the first four weeks of the study. Those individuals who continued on the drug had lost seven pounds on average at one year. By the end of the second year there was regaining of some of the weight, but it was clearly better than the placebo group— the average weight loss was about five pounds. Only about one-third of the people who entered the study were still participating at the end of the two years. Orlistat does appear to have a favorable effect on lipids: it lowers triglycerides, total cholesterol, and LDL cholesterol.

Orlistat can impair the absorption of fat-soluble vitamins A, D, E, and K, so if you take Orlistat, take a vitamin supplement containing these vitamins.

RIMONABANT (ACOMPLIA)

Rimonabant is an antagonist; that is, it prevents the CB1 receptor from being stimulated and reduces appetite. Over a one-year period, patients on 20 mg of rimonabant had an eleven-pound weight loss, and when followed for a second year maintained the weight loss, whereas those who came off the drug regained the weight. The main side effects were nausea, anxiety, and depression. About 40 percent of the subjects did not complete the trial. It is too early to say how useful this medication will be in helping weight control.

Bariatric Surgery:
Surgery to Promote Weight Loss

When bariatric surgery is performed in people with type 2 diabetes, 60 percent or more have normal blood glucose levels without medications, and the others can use fewer medications. There is also improvement in the lipid profile, blood pressure, and sleep apnea. The National Institutes of Health recommend that bariatric surgery is one option that should be considered if a person has extreme obesity (BMI greater than 40) or if a person has diabetes and a BMI greater than 35.

There are two kinds of bariatric surgeries that are performed for weight loss:

- In restrictive surgery the size of the stomach is reduced by using an adjustable gastric band, cinched around the stomach like a belt.

- In malabsorptive surgery the food is diverted so that it does not get absorbed as effectively. The Roux-en-Y gastric bypass procedure is currently the most popular procedure—a small stomach pouch is created

DID YOU KNOW?

The CB1 Receptor

Apart from its effect of causing euphoria, marijuana (or cannabis) also increases appetite—what is described as "the munchies." Marijuana works on receptors in the brain called CB1 receptors, thus stimulating eating. So researchers used this idea to see whether the opposite could be true: could a medication work on the CB1 receptors to discourage eating? Rimonabant is the first of such medicines.

and separated from the rest of the stomach, and the outlet of this newly created pouch empties into the lower part of the small intestine and so causes malabsorption.

A year after the Roux-en-Y gastric bypass procedure, patients have lost over 75 percent of their excess weight. There is some regaining of the weight, but the weight loss is still 50 to 60 percent of excess weight at ten years or more. The adjustable gastric banding procedure initially results in less weight loss. During the course of a three-year study, most patients had lost an average of 36 percent of their excess weight.

Clearly, bariatric surgery is the most effective therapy we have for type 2 diabetes. The surgery is now done with laparoscopes, and the risk of death is less than 1 percent. However, there are a number of side effects. The adjustable gastric banding can cause nausea and vomiting, heartburn, and abdominal pain. The band can slip, so some people may need a second surgery. The Roux-en-Y gastric bypass operation impairs absorption of nutrients. Impaired absorption of iron and vitamin B_{12} can cause anemia, and impaired calcium absorption can cause bone loss. Therefore, people who have this procedure must take iron, calcium, and vitamin supplements. Some people can also get a "dumping syndrome" due to the rapid emptying of the stomach contents into the intestine, causing nausea, sweating, faintness, and diarrhea after eating. This can be quite disabling. Occasionally, they can get reactive hypoglycemia, with glucose levels in the 30s to 40s after a carbohydrate-rich meal.

Summary

- There is good evidence that combined intervention of a low-calorie diet, behavioral therapy, and increased physical activity provide the best weight-loss and weight-maintenance results.

- High-protein, low-carbohydrate, and low-fat diets do work, but in the long term they are no more effective than conventional diets. Long-term safety of the high-protein, low-carbohydrate diets is lacking. Very low calorie diets can cause weight loss over the short term, but the weight goes up over the subsequent one to two years.

- Medications for weight loss are only modestly effective, and their main use is in conjunction with diet and exercise weight-loss interventions. The weight is regained once the drugs are stopped.

- Bariatric surgery is the most effective weight-loss approach, but there are side effects from the surgery. At this time it may only be appropriate for those people with a BMI greater than 35 who, despite their best efforts, are not able to lose weight, whose diabetes is not well controlled, and who are developing complications.

PART THREE

Additional Considerations

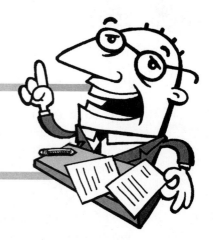

CHAPTER 11

Managing Your Diabetes While Traveling

With proper planning, there is no problem traveling with diabetes. The things you need to think about and plan for include the following:

- Managing diabetes supplies
- Diabetes management during your flight
- Adjusting insulin for time changes
- Managing diabetes complications
- Avoiding and/or treating traveler's illnesses, especially gastroenteritis

Managing Diabetes Supplies

Take adequate supplies for your diabetes management when you travel. In fact, take twice the amount of diabetes medication and supplies that you will normally need.

If you are on an insulin pump (see Chapter 6), take some basal insulin such as insulin glargine and syringes in case you have a pump failure. Keep the insulin cool by packing it in an insulated bag with refrigerated gel packs, or use Frio packs (see friouk.com/index.php).

Also take glucose tablets, gels, and snacks for treatment of hypoglycemia and a glucagon kit and ketone testing strips. Ideally, take two glucose meters and pack them in separate bags. Keep most of your supplies in your carry-on luggage, but keep some supplies in your checked luggage, just in case you lose your carry-on luggage.

Some health insurance companies will only fill your prescriptions with one month's supply of medicines at a time, but if you call ahead, they will usually authorize an additional supply with a "vacation override."

You should also carry a travel letter from your doctor explaining that you have type 1 or 2 diabetes and the medications you are using to treat it. This note should also include the medicines you are taking for other conditions as well as any food and drug allergies you have. Also obtain a spare prescription for all your medications in case you lose your supplies or your stay is prolonged. Wear your MedicAlert bracelet at all times, and carry a card or letter explaining that you have diabetes written in the languages of the places you are visiting. Keep a list of emergency phone numbers: your doctor's office, your pharmacy, your insulin pump company, and (if you're traveling abroad) the American embassy or consulate and a list of English-speaking doctors in the country you are visiting. The International Diabetes Federation website (see Resources) has contact information for diabetes organizations in many countries.

If you are traveling by airplane and are concerned about new (and ever-changing) regulations concerning fluids in your carry-on bag, call the airline well in advance of your flight.

Diabetes Management on the Airplane

If food will not be served on your flight, take food and fast-acting carbohydrate with you. If it is a long flight with a meal (and keep in mind that in-flight meals are rare these days), it is not necessary to order a special meal on the plane, but it is a good idea to have some food with you (two to three snacks) in case the meal is delayed. Inject your insulin dose *after* your meal arrives. Since the pressure in an airplane is different than the pressure on the ground, do not inject air into the vial before drawing up your insulin into the syringe. Check your blood glucose frequently during the flight. You may need a little more insulin because you are inactive. If you are traveling alone and are concerned that you might experience hypoglycemia, tell the flight attendants that you have diabetes so they can keep an eye on you.

Drink plenty of fluids during the flight. Wear loose-fitting shoes because your feet might swell, and walk around the airplane when possible and do some leg-stretching exercises to avoid blood clots.

Adjusting Your Insulin for Time Changes

The body's sensitivity to insulin varies throughout the day and night. You are most insulin sensitive early in the night and most resistant early in the morning. These changes in insulin sensitivity are due to the daily fluctuations in the levels of hormones, particularly cortisol. The internal body clock that regulates these hormones gets cues from environmental light and temperature. When you go to a different time zone, the body clock and the hormones reset to the new light-dark cycle. This resetting process takes time and explains why you feel "jet-lagged." The challenge for people who are on insulin is to figure out how to adjust basal insulin levels while the body is getting used to being in the new time zone. The solution is to make sure that you have a safe basal rate and to use bolus insulin doses to cover any high blood glucose levels:

- If the time zone adjustment is only one to three hours, ignore it and just give the basal insulin at your usual time in the new time zone. For example, if you give your insulin glargine at 10 P.M., then do so at 10 P.M. in the new time zone.

- If you travel east (shorter day) and the time zone change is long, give bolus insulin every four hours and delay giving the basal insulin until at least twenty-four hours have passed since the last basal insulin injection.

- If you are traveling west (longer day), inject bolus insulin every four hours until you inject your basal insulin at your usual time in the new time zone.

- If you are on a pump, you can change the pump clock to the new time. If the time zone change is long, you may go on the lowest basal rate until the jet lag has resolved and then you can set up new basal doses.

Since activity and diet may be different when you are traveling, you may have to adjust your basal insulin even if the time difference is negligible.

Managing Diabetes Complications

If you have other diseases associated with diabetes, keep the following in mind as you travel:

- Protect your feet if you have peripheral neuropathy and loss of protective threshold. Take walking shoes that you know will work for you rather than buying new shoes for the trip. Limit the amount of walking you do if you have significant foot deformities.

- If you have autonomic neuropathy, make sure that you drink plenty of fluids to avoid getting light-headed.

- If you have heart disease, be careful not to overexert yourself.

- Continue taking all your medications as prescribed.

- Avoid too much sun exposure, especially if you are taking oral medications for your diabetes.

Preventing Illness While Traveling

Get the appropriate immunizations and take the usual precautions to avoid getting ill (see Resources). Take antinausea (prochlorperazine) and antidiarrheal (loperamide) medications and a supply of antibiotics with you. If you do get sick, the sick day rules apply (see Chapter 12).

Summary

- Take twice as much of your medicines and diabetes supplies as you will use.

- Carry a letter from your doctor that explains that you have diabetes and lists your medicines and allergies.

- When adjusting insulin for time zone changes, the most important thing to remember is not to give a basal insulin injection until the effect of the previous basal injection has worn off.

- Changes in diet and activity will impact your glucose levels, and therefore you will need to review your glucose levels frequently and adjust your diabetes medicines as necessary.

- Take extra precautions if you have complications of diabetes.

- Follow the CDC guidelines for safe travel. Have a backup plan for what to do if you fall sick.

CHAPTER 12

Managing Diabetes While Sick and During Medical Procedures and Hospitalization

When you have diabetes and also develop another illness, you must take extra precautions. When you are ill, a number of different factors will impact your glucose control:

- Your body's stress hormones rise, and this can raise your glucose levels unless you adjust your diabetes medications appropriately.

- Being less active while ill can raise your glucose levels.

- You may not eat as much, so you may need less diabetes medication for the food.

- Medicines that you take for your illness may affect your glucose levels— for example, prednisone for an asthma attack.

How should you adjust your diabetes medications when you are sick? This chapter tells you how. I also discuss what to do if you find yourself hospitalized.

What to Do if You Get Sick and Are on Insulin

Do not stop your insulin—depending on the severity of the illness you may need the same or more insulin. If you have type 1 diabetes and you stop the insulin, you will go into DKA (see Chapter 3). If you are on a basal-bolus insulin regimen, take the same amount of the long-acting insulin as you normally do. If you are on a pump, keep the basal rates the same. Cover your carbohydrates with insulin in the usual way. If you have vomiting and you are not sure if you will keep the food down, you can give the insulin for the carbohydrates afterward. Correct any high glucose levels with fast-acting insulin analogs.

If you have type 2 diabetes and are on premixed insulins twice a day, you may take the same amount of insulin *if* you know that you can keep some food down. If you are not sure that you will be able to eat, check with your doctor—you may need to cut back on your premixed insulin to 50 to 75 percent of the dose.

Be sure to also do the following:

- Check the blood glucose frequently—every two to four hours.

- Drink plenty of fluids: sips of water, diet soda, sugar-free lemonade, sugar-free Popsicles, and broth are all acceptable.

- If you cannot eat solid foods, drink juices, regular sodas, or Gatorade or eat Jell-O.

- Check ketones—either in the urine or in the blood—at least once or twice a day.

- It is fine to take over-the-counter cough medicines: don't worry about the sugar in these medicines.

- Contact your medical team (see Chapter 4) or go to the emergency room if you cannot keep down fluids, if your blood glucose levels remain high (more than 250) despite taking extra insulin, if you have high levels of ketones in blood or urine, or if you have abdominal pain, shortness of breath, or sleepiness.

- For children who cannot keep down carbohydrates and whose glucose is getting low, the parent can give a glucagon injection (see Chapter 14).

If You Get Sick and Are on Oral Diabetes Medicines or Exenatide

If you are able to eat and keep down food, you can take your usual oral medications or exenatide injections for the diabetes. If you have significant nausea and vomiting, call your doctor to get specific instructions—for example, you may need to hold off on the exenatide injections. Sometimes illnesses significantly raise the glucose levels and the oral medications are not very effective. In this case, you may need some insulin temporarily.

Drink plenty of fluids, and if you cannot eat solid foods drink juices, regular sodas, and broth.

Monitor blood glucose levels frequently—every four to six hours.

Managing Your Diabetes During Medical Procedures and Hospitalizations

Having an outpatient medical procedure or being hospitalized can be a stressful experience. Planning for it can alleviate some of the stress and ensure that your diabetes is well managed. In this section, I discuss how to adjust medicines for procedures that require you not to eat and how to talk to medical providers about your

DID YOU KNOW?

Avoiding Sickness

Having diabetes can complicate the management of common illnesses such as the flu, so all people with diabetes should get a flu shot every year. The pneumococcal vaccine is normally given to people over age sixty-five, but if you have diabetes and you are over eighteen years old, you should also get a pneumococcal vaccine to reduce the risk of one type of pneumonia.

diabetes before the procedure or hospitalization, tell you what to take with you when you go into the hospital, and let you know how you can ensure that your diabetes remains under control during the hospitalization and afterwards.

OUTPATIENT PROCEDURES

Many medical procedures, such as colonoscopies, hernia repair, cataracts, cosmetic surgeries, and x-ray procedures such as angiograms are performed in an outpatient setting, where you go into the hospital in the morning and leave a few hours after the procedure.

If you need one of these procedures, talk to your medical care team beforehand about how to manage your diabetes. A lot of these procedures require you not to eat for several hours before and after the procedure. Therefore, you need to know how to adjust your diabetes medicines to avoid both low and high glucose levels. Ideally, the procedure should be scheduled early in the day so that your period of fasting is limited. There are also issues surrounding diabetes-related complications—gastroparesis can become troublesome and can cause vomiting after the procedure. The contrast dyes used in x-rays can worsen kidney function, especially if you already have diabetic kidney disease.

The following are general recommendations for what to do regarding your diabetes medicines before, during, and after the procedure. Your medical team will provide specific recommendations.

If You Take Oral Medicines

In most cases you can take your usual medicines the day before the procedure, but none on the day of the procedure, and then restart them when you start eating. If you are on metformin and you need a procedure where you get a special x-ray with contrast dye, you may be asked to stop your metformin for a couple of days until a serum creatine confirms that your kidneys are not affected by the contrast dye. When you stop metformin, your glucose levels may run high, and your doctor may ask you to take tolbutamide, repaglinide, or nateglinide, or even a little bit of insulin, to control the glucose levels until you can restart the metformin.

If You Take Insulin

In most cases, you can take your usual insulin dose the day before surgery. How much insulin is injected on the day of the surgery will depend on your particular insulin regimen. Let me give you some scenarios:

- **If you are on a basal-bolus insulin regimen**—that is, you are using insulin glargine at night and a fast-acting insulin analog before meals—then you should continue your insulin glargine (perhaps reducing the dose just a little bit—about 10 percent) while fasting, and use fast-acting insulin to correct high glucose levels. For example, if you are going to get a colonoscopy: the day before the procedure, use fast-acting insulin for the liquid carbohydrates you consume and take your usual insulin glargine that night. On the day of the colonoscopy, do not take any fast-acting insulin until you have recovered from the procedure and are ready to eat.

- **If you are on a premixed insulin regimen,** inject the usual insulin dose the day before the procedure. On the day of the procedure, your insulin dose will depend on your glucose levels and what happens if you miss an insulin injection. If your glucose levels tend to go up a lot if you miss an injection and do not eat, then you will need to take some insulin. On the other hand, if your glucose does not rise much if you do not eat and do not take insulin, then you can probably wait and hold off the insulin injection until after the procedure. Usually, you can restart the insulin with the evening meal. If you are going to eat less than usual that evening, cut back the insulin dose.

- **If you are on an insulin pump,** switch to insulin injections a couple of days before the procedure, because while you are undergoing the procedure, the pump infusion cannula can get dislodged, interrupting the insulin flow. Also, the medical personnel who are looking after you may not be familiar with how to manage a pump. To come off the pump, just calculate the total amount of basal insulin you take in twenty-four hours and give that amount of insulin as one injection of insulin glargine. For example, if you are on a basal rate of 0.5 units per hour, then the total basal in twenty-four hours is $24 \times 0.5 = 12$ units. Take 12 units of insulin glargine and turn off the pump. Remember that insulin glargine takes a couple of hours to start working, so you may need to give a small bolus of your fast-acting insulin (1 to 2 units) to cover this two-hour interval.

PLANNED HOSPITALIZATION

To get optimal treatment for your diabetes when you have a planned admission to the hospital for medical or surgical treatment, you need to consider the following.

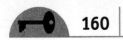

Before Going to the Hospital

Talk to your prospective medical team about your diabetes management while in the hospital:

- Who will be involved in managing your diabetes? Does the hospital have a diabetes nurse specialist?

- Are you going to stay on your oral medicines, or will they switch you to insulin injections for the duration of your stay?

- What about meals: how long before you can eat normally?

- When you leave the hospital, will you be able to go back to your regular medicines, or will you require insulin for a short time?

- Can you use your insulin pump in the hospital? If not, you should switch to a basal-bolus insulin injection regimen a few days before you go in.

Talk to your family members about your diabetes and keep them involved so they can be your advocates if you cannot speak for yourself. Take the following things with you to the hospital:

- Several copies of a list of all your medicines—the doses and how often you take them; your insulin regimen, including the scale you use to adjust for high glucose levels; and any known food or drug allergies (take several copies because almost invariably, the doctor or nurse will misplace your first copy)

- The bottles of all your medicines

- A list of all your previous illnesses and when they occurred

- Your diet at home: how many grams of carbohydrate you usually eat at each meal

- Your diabetes kit, including your blood glucose monitor and lancet device, blood glucose strips, glucose log, glucose tablets, insulin syringes, and your insulin vial or pen

- Insulin pump supplies if you are going to use your pump in the hospital

- Your MedicAlert bracelet

- Your advanced health directive: this gives your medical team guidance about what kind of care should be given to you if you cannot make decisions for yourself, and the name of the person whom you designate to make health decisions on your behalf

While You Are in the Hospital

Glucose management in the hospital can be challenging for a number of reasons:

- The stress of the illness or operation can raise your blood glucose, and the doses of the diabetes medicines you normally use may not be sufficient to control the glucose rise.

- There may be altered schedules of eating and activity in the hospital. You might have to be fasting for various procedures; food may arrive at different times; you may not want to eat because of your illness; and the food is different from what you are used to.

- The oral diabetes medicines may have to be stopped because they may not be safe to use while you are ill, and you will be switched over to insulin during the hospital stay because it can be rapidly adjusted to meet your altering needs.

If you have type 1 diabetes or you have type 2 diabetes and are on insulin and you are not going to eat for twenty-four hours or more, you may be given insulin and fluids into the vein (an insulin infusion) to keep your glucose under control. The nurse will adjust the insulin infusion based on finger-stick blood glucose tests performed every one to two hours. The infusion is continued until you are eating, and then you will be switched to subcutaneous injections.

The usual insulin regimen is a fast-acting insulin before meals, and if insulin is needed overnight, either NPH, insulin detemir, or insulin glargine at bedtime. A small correction of fast-acting insulin might also be needed at bedtime and 2 A.M. People with type 2 diabetes can sometimes be given premixed insulin twice daily.

To help keep your glucose levels under control while in the hospital, do the following:

- Keep your diabetes kit nearby so you can check your glucose if you need to. Also ask the medical care team if you can have glucose tablets or juice available in case you have a hypoglycemic reaction.

- Ask to see the nutritionist and explain your diet plan to him or her so that you can get the meals that you desire.

- If the hospital has a diabetes nurse specialist, work with him or her to troubleshoot problems.

- Work with the nurses on the timing and dosing of your diabetes medicines. If your food arrives but the nurse has not come by to give your insulin injection, you should call the nurse to give your injection before eating.

Also, if you know that your appetite is not normal, eat the carbohydrate foods first. If you are not sure that you will be able to keep any food down, ask the nurse to let you eat first and then give you your fast-acting insulin analog.

- Keep talking to your medical team about your glucose control, and request an endocrine consultation if your diabetes control is proving difficult to manage.

As you recover and are getting ready to go home, your medical team may switch you back to your usual diabetes medicines. However, if it looks like you are going to stay on insulin, the inpatient diabetes team—the diabetes nurse specialist, pharmacist, and nutritionist—will teach you how to count carbohydrates and how to inject and adjust insulin.

When You Are Discharged from the Hospital

Before you leave the hospital, talk to the pharmacist or diabetes nurse specialist and make sure that you know how to take your diabetes medicines and how often to check your blood glucose levels. If you are on insulin, know how to adjust the insulin as your food intake and activity changes and what to do when you have low or high glucose values. You should also know whom to call if there are problems.

After discharge, schedule an appointment with your primary care physician to review your diabetes management.

EMERGENCY HOSPITALIZATION

Even though you cannot know when an emergency will happen, you can plan ahead. Make plans for an unexpected hospitalization by doing the following:

- Always keep an updated list of your medicines, including doses, in your wallet and wear your MedicAlert bracelet.

- If you are on insulin or oral diabetes medicines that can cause low blood glucose reactions, you should have your diabetes kit with you at all times.

- When you are admitted to the emergency room, make sure that the medical staff members know you have diabetes.

- Keep contact information for family members or friends in your wallet.

- If you are in the emergency room for a long time, have the emergency room nurses check your blood glucose levels from time to time. If you are not feeling well, keep asking until you get help.

- Talk to your next of kin before any such event, and let them know where you keep your medicines and diabetes supplies at home and where your durable power of attorney form for health care is kept so that you can have them bring these to the hospital.

Summary

- When you are sick:
  - Keep taking your diabetes medicines, but you may need to adjust the doses.
  - Check your blood glucose levels frequently.
  - Drink plenty of fluids.
  - Check for ketones if you have type 1 diabetes and have nausea and vomiting.
- When you have to fast for medical procedures:
  - Talk to your diabetes care team about how to manage your glucose when you need to fast for medical procedures.
  - If you have type 1 diabetes, you should take your basal insulin but not the bolus insulin before the procedure.
  - If you have type 2 diabetes, you can usually wait until after the procedure before restarting the diabetes medicines.
- When you have to go into the hospital, do the following:
  - Make sure that the treating doctors and nurses know about your diabetes and how you treat it.
  - Involve family members so that if you are incapacitated, they can advocate for you.

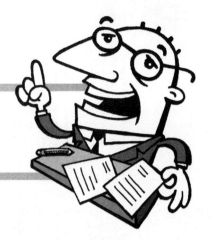

CHAPTER 13

Diabetes and Pregnancy

Diabetes complicates about 8 percent of pregnancies each year. About 75 percent of these diabetic pregnancies are gestational diabetes—that is, the woman is diagnosed as having diabetes during the pregnancy. Of the remaining, 23 percent involve preexisting type 2 diabetes and about 1 to 2 percent involves preexisting type 1 diabetes.

The issues surrounding preexisting diabetes are slightly different from those faced by women who first develop diabetes during pregnancy. Women who have diabetes before they become pregnant have to deal with glucose control at conception and early in pregnancy. If there are any diabetes-related complications, these may also have an impact on the pregnancy. Women who have gestational diabetes are faced with learning all about diabetes, including watching their diet and taking insulin, while pregnant. This chapter gives you details on both situations.

Planning Pregnancy with Preexisting Diabetes

Women with preexisting diabetes face a number of issues, which are discussed in the following sections.

FERTILITY

Recent studies suggest that fertility in women with type 1 diabetes is the same as in women without diabetes. Polycystic ovary syndrome (PCOS) is a risk factor for type 2 diabetes, and women with this condition may have difficulty with ovulation and getting pregnant. Metformin, pioglitazone, and rosiglitazone can make the menstrual cycles regular and cause ovulation in women with polycystic ovary syndrome. Metformin is frequently used for this purpose, and the medication is stopped when the woman becomes pregnant.

Keep in mind that men with type 1 diabetes who have neurological complications can have problems with erections and ejaculation. It is still unclear whether diabetes affects sperm motility and semen volume in men with diabetes.

PRECONCEPTION ASSESSMENT AND CONTROL

If you are a woman with diabetes, you should plan your pregnancies and attend a high-risk obstetric practice to get preconception counseling to learn about the following:

- The risk of your child developing diabetes
- The blood glucose targets you should aim for before conception and during pregnancy
- The impact of complications of diabetes (retinopathy, kidney disease, heart disease, and neuropathy) on the pregnancy
- Nutrition during pregnancy
- Monitoring of the developing fetus

In the following sections, I talk about each of these counseling points briefly.

The Risk of Your Child Developing Diabetes

Prospective parents may be fearful of transmitting diabetes to their children. The risk of transmitting type 1 diabetes is quite low (6 percent if the father has type 1 diabetes and 3 percent if the mother has type 1 diabetes). The risk of transmitting the genetic risk is higher in type 2 diabetes: if the mother has type 2 diabetes, the risk is about 18 percent, increasing to 50 percent if both parents have type 2 diabetes. The environment, however, plays a bigger role in the development of type 2 diabetes, regardless of the genetic risk.

Blood Glucose Control

Table 13-1 lists the glucose targets that you should aim for immediately before and during pregnancy.

You will need to monitor your blood glucose levels frequently—before each meal, one and a half to two hours after a meal, at bedtime, and at 2 A.M. Additional checks may be necessary if you are driving. Poor glucose control at conception increases the risk of spontaneous abortion and of congenital malformations of the heart, kidney, nervous system, or skeleton. Controlling the diabetes so that the HbA1c is normal before and early during pregnancy reduces the risk of these congenital malformations. Table 13-2 shows the risks of congenital malformations in relation to HbA1c levels (see Chapter 5).

Good blood glucose control remains important even later in the pregnancy. High glucose levels can cause a number of problems:

- Polyhydramnios, a term used to describe too much amniotic fluid, which can lead to premature labor

- Stillbirth

- A large fetus due to high fetal insulin in response to the high maternal glucose. This condition is referred to as **macrosomia**. Labor can be complicated with such a large fetus, and a cesarean section may be necessary. Babies with macrosomia are likely to have low blood glucose reactions after birth, they may not feed well, and they may have breathing problems, low calcium levels, and jaundice.

- Ketoacidosis is very serious during pregnancy and can lead to fetal death.

- It is also important not to be overaggressive in controlling the glucose levels—if postmeal glucose levels are not allowed to rise at all, there may be insufficient fetal growth, leading to a "small for dates" infant.

Complications of Diabetes

Two aspects of diabetes complications need to be considered when a woman is contemplating pregnancy. First, there is the impact of the pregnancy on diabetic com-

Table 13-1 Glucose Targets During Pregnancy	
Fasting and premeal blood glucose levels	60 to 100 mg/dl
Peak glucose levels after meals	Less than 130 mg/dl
Bedtime and 2 A.M. glucose levels	100 mg/dl

Table 13-2 Risk of Fetal Malformation with Elevated HbA1c	
HbA1c Level	**Fetal Malformation Rate**
Less than 6% is normal	
Less than 6.9%	No increase in rate
7 to 8.5%	5%
Greater than 10%	22.4%

Source: Miller E, Hare JW, Cloherty JP, Dunn PJ, Gleason RE, Soeldner JS, Kitzmiller JL. "Elevated maternal hemoglobin A1c in early pregnancy and major congenital anomalies in infants of diabetic mothers." *N Engl J Med* 1981 May 28; 304 (22): 1331–34.

plications and maternal health, and second, the effects of diabetic complications on fetal health.

- **Diabetic retinopathy:** New diabetic retinopathy can suddenly appear during pregnancy, and retinopathy that is already present can get worse. There are two possible reasons for the deterioration: First, if your diabetes control has been poor and you suddenly tighten it over a short period of time (such as getting ready for pregnancy), the rapid improvement itself can cause a flare-up of the retinopathy. Second, the hormonal and circulatory changes that occur in pregnancy may worsen the retinopathy. If you have significant retinopathy before you become pregnant, you might require treatment during the pregnancy. Therefore, you will need to see an ophthalmologist before and during the pregnancy. The retinopathy usually improves after the pregnancy.

- **Diabetic kidney disease:** If you have kidney disease secondary to your diabetes, pregnancy can make the kidney disease worse. Often the kidney disease will recover after delivery, but it may not if the prepregnancy kidney failure is more severe. Women with diabetic kidney disease who are contemplating pregnancy should therefore consider getting an opinion from a nephrologist (kidney doctor).

- **Preeclampsia:** Preeclampsia is a serious condition where there is severe elevation in blood pressure, fluid retention, and protein loss. It occurs more often in women with diabetes. About 15 to 45 percent of women with diabetes who have microalbuminuria (see Chapter 3) develop preeclampsia. Hospitalization and early delivery may be necessary.

- **Blood pressure medications:** If you are taking ACE inhibitors to control your blood pressure, your doctor will switch you to other blood pressure medicines because ACE inhibitors cannot be taken during pregnancy.

• **Heart disease:** During pregnancy, there is increase in blood volume and blood flow, and this causes the heart rate to go up. A normal heart handles this increased demand without any problems, but it can be a problem in women with heart disease. The risk of heart disease is higher in women with long-standing, poorly controlled type 2 diabetes who also have high lipid levels and high blood pressure; and in women with type 1 diabetes who have multiple complications with autonomic neuropathy and kidney disease. If you have any of these risk factors for heart disease, you should get an evaluation from a cardiologist before becoming pregnant.

• **Lipid therapy:** The FDA has not approved cholesterol-lowering medicines for use during pregnancy, and if you are taking any of these drugs, you should discontinue them. Women with diabetes who have high triglyceride levels can develop pancreatitis during pregnancy. Therefore, if you have high triglycerides before you become pregnant, you should work with your nutritionist to take whatever measures are necessary to lower the triglycerides.

• **Thyroid disease:** You should be screened for thyroid disease before becoming pregnant. If you are hypothyroid, your thyroid hormone replacement medication will need dose adjustments during pregnancy.

• **Gastroparesis:** In the first trimester, diabetic gastroparesis can worsen the nausea and vomiting of pregnancy, and sometimes women will need to be admitted to a hospital for intravenous fluids and nutrition because they get dehydrated and malnourished. Occasionally this problem continues throughout the pregnancy.

Treatment of Diabetes During Pregnancy

Although there is evidence that oral glyburide is safe in pregnancy, the current practice is to have women control their diabetes with insulin when they are pregnant. If you have type 2 diabetes and you are using oral agents for your diabetes, you will be switched over to insulin before you start trying to get pregnant. Not all insulins, however, are approved for use during pregnancy. The fast-acting insulin analogs insulin lispro and insulin aspart are safe. Currently, the only long-acting insulin used during pregnancy is NPH. Recently, a small study of insulin glargine used in thirty-two pregnancies did not show any problems. There is no information about using insulin detemir during pregnancy.

The goal of treatment is to get your HbA1c level into the normal range before you try to get pregnant. The time it takes to do this varies, so you may want to plan at least three months to achieve this. You may need to visit your diabetes team every two to three weeks during this time.

Once you have stable glucose levels in the target range, with a normal HbA1c, then you can try to get pregnant. Once you are pregnant, your care will be transitioned to a specialty high-risk obstetrics practice staffed by a team that consists of an obstetrician, a nutritionist, a diabetes educator, a nurse, and an endocrinologist.

Your insulin doses will vary during the pregnancy due to the hormonal changes. At about nine to twelve weeks you may need slightly less insulin, but then the insulin doses usually will go up until about thirty-six weeks.

NUTRITION

During pregnancy, you should have a balanced diet of 40 to 50 percent of calories as carbohydrate, 20 percent protein, and 30 to 40 percent fat. The number of calories you can take will depend on your prepregnancy weight: approximately 13.5 kcal per pound per day (30 kcal/kg/day) if you are currently at your ideal weight; 11 kcal per pound per day (24 kcal/kg/day) if you are 20 to 50 percent above your ideal weight, and 5.5 to 8 kcal per pound per day (12 to 18 kcal/kg/day) if you are more than 50 percent above your ideal body weight (1 kg equals 2.2 pounds). For more on a balanced diet, see Chapter 8.

FETAL SURVEILLANCE

As with most pregnancies, ultrasound is used with diabetic women to follow the development of the fetus. It allows the obstetrician to estimate the age, growth, and health of the fetus and to look for malformations.

LABOR AND DELIVERY

With careful management of the diabetes in pregnancy, most women are able to go to term unless there are complications. Generally speaking, pregnancies are not allowed to proceed beyond forty weeks.

If you have type 1 diabetes, you will be given an intravenous infusion of insulin and glucose to keep your glucose levels between 70 and 90 mg/dl during labor and delivery. High glucose levels can increase the risk of hypoglycemia in the fetus. During the active part of labor, the insulin may be stopped and a glucose infusion may be required to supply the mother with calories. After delivery, your doctor will change you back to your prepregnancy insulin doses.

If you have type 2 diabetes, your doctor may ask you to stay on insulin while you are breast-feeding, and once you stop, he or she will switch you to your usual medicines for glucose control.

Gestational Diabetes

During pregnancy, women are screened for diabetes at twenty-four to twenty-eight weeks, or at the very first visit if they are at very high risk of diabetes as indicated by the following risk factors:

- There are family members with diabetes.
- Her ethnic background is a group that is particularly susceptible to diabetes.
- She has polycystic ovarian syndrome.
- She had diabetes with a previous pregnancy or delivered a baby weighing more than nine pounds.

There are two tests that can determine whether a woman has gestational diabetes. The first test is performed on all non-high-risk women at the twenty-four to twenty-eight week visit. If this test is normal, no further testing is necessary. If this first test is positive, however, a second test is performed about a week later.

- **First test: One-hour 50-gram glucose challenge screening test.** In this test you take a drink that contains 50 grams of glucose (there is no need to fast beforehand). The blood glucose level is checked after one hour. If your glucose level is greater than 130 mg/dl, the test is positive. If the glucose level is 180 mg/dl or more, there is a strong likelihood that you have diabetes and you will be asked to do a fasting glucose test. Then, if this fasting glucose test is 126 mg/dl or greater, you have gestational diabetes.

- **Second test: Three-hour 100-gram glucose test.** If the 50-gram glucose challenge test is positive, then within one week you will do a fasting three-hour 100-gram glucose test (see Table 13-3). You should eat your usual diet, including carbohydrates, in the days before the test—in other words, don't change your eating habits and stop eating carbohydrates in the days between the first and second test—and fast for eight to fourteen hours before taking the test. The second test is considered positive for diabetes if two or more values are at or above the threshold levels. If only one value is abnormal, this test will be repeated in four weeks.

Table 13-3	Three-Hour 100-Gram Glucose Test
Fasting	95 mg/dl
1 hour	180 mg/dl
2 hours	155 mg/dl
3 hours	140 mg/dl

Source: Coustan DR, Carpenter MW. "The diagnosis of gestational diabetes." *Diabetes Care* 1998 Aug; 21 (Suppl 2): B5–8.

TREATMENT

After you are diagnosed with gestational diabetes, you will be taught how to check your blood glucose at home, especially your postprandial (after meals) glucose levels. You will also meet a nutritionist to work out a meal plan or diet. If your glucose levels are not normal on the diet—that is, over 90 mg/dl fasting, more than 130 mg/dl after meals—then you will start insulin therapy, although glyburide therapy can be considered.

LABOR AND DELIVERY

Women with gestational diabetes are usually allowed to go into spontaneous labor. Depending on the glucose levels, you may need insulin during the labor. Usually insulin is not required after delivery.

GESTATIONAL DIABETES AND RISK FOR TYPE 2 NONGESTATIONAL DIABETES

If you have gestational diabetes, your risk of developing type 2 diabetes in the future is 5 to 50 percent. Therefore, you should have a two-hour 75-gram oral glucose tolerance test (OGTT) six to ten weeks after delivery.

Summary

- With tight glucose control and careful management of diabetes complications, women with diabetes can have healthy babies:
  - Optimal glucose control before conception and early in pregnancy reduces the risk of fetal malformations.

- Later in pregnancy, tight glucose control reduces the risk of macrosomia and stillbirth.

- Diabetes complications can impact maternal and fetal health during the pregnancy:

  - Retinopathy can progress during pregnancy, and you should see an ophthalmologist before and during pregnancy.

  - Kidney disease can also progress during pregnancy, and its presence increases the risk for preeclampsia.

- Gestational diabetes is diabetes that first appears during the pregnancy.

  - If diet does not normalize the glucose levels, insulin therapy should be initiated.

  - Usually gestational diabetes resolves after the pregnancy, but these women are at higher risk for developing type 2 diabetes in the future.

  - Maintaining normal weight and exercising regularly may delay or prevent the onset of diabetes in women who have had gestational diabetes.

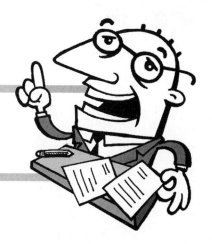

CHAPTER 14

When Your Child Has Diabetes

About 50 percent of new cases of type 1 diabetes occur in childhood and adolescence. In fact, over the past twenty years, type 1 diabetes has been occurring earlier in childhood. There has also been an increase in the incidence of type 2 diabetes in childhood. As with diabetes in adults, it is important to distinguish between type 1 and type 2 diabetes because the treatments of the two types are different.

Your Role as a Parent

When you discover that your child has diabetes, you will probably be very upset. Being a parent is hard work in the best of circumstances, and your child's diabetes will add a whole other dimension to being a parent. You will need to learn everything you can about diabetes in addition to all your other parenting duties. This may be overwhelming, but with patience and perseverance and the support of your child's diabetes care team, you will be able to help your child manage the disease so that he or she can have the disease but still do all a child needs to do. Your child's diabetes care team (ideally a pediatric endocrinologist, diabetes educator, nutritionist, and psychologist) will help you, your child, and your family learn the following survival skills for managing the diabetes:

- How to monitor the glucose levels
- How to recognize and treat low and high glucose levels
- How to adjust insulin and/or oral medications for foods and exercise
- How to treat the diabetes when your child is ill
- How to involve other family members, other caregivers, and the staff at your child's school
- How to transfer responsibilities as your child grows up

Type 1 Diabetes

The symptoms that lead to a diagnosis of type 1 diabetes in children include the following:

- Weight loss with either increased appetite or loss of appetite (more common in the younger child)
- Increased thirst
- Increased urination: a toilet-trained child may start wetting, or a baby in diapers will need more frequent changes
- Dehydration
- Severe diaper rash that does not respond to the usual treatment
- Vomiting that is persistent, particularly if it is accompanied by weakness or drowsiness

CHALLENGES AT DIFFERENT AGES

You and your child will face unique challenges as he or she ages.

Infants Less than One Year Old

In infants, your biggest challenge is recognizing hypoglycemia—your child may be sweaty or restless or pale. Therefore, it is important to monitor the glucose levels frequently, maybe even during the night. The goal is not to achieve normal glucose levels, but to avoid very high and very low glucose values.

Toddlers—Ages One to Three

With toddlers, it is best to establish a schedule with food and insulin injections. This can be challenging, especially with a child who refuses to eat or is a picky eater. Hypoglycemia is the biggest concern with this age group, and often it is best managed by giving insulin after a meal. Other steps that you can take include the following:

- Establish a routine for checking glucose and injections.
- Use a glucose meter that requires the smallest blood sample and gives quick results.
- Test glucose levels on arms, where it hurts less than at fingertips (see Chapter 5).

Children—Ages Three to Seven

Quite often, children this age participate in their diabetes management by helping with glucose monitoring and choosing foods. This is also the age when parents will need to involve other caregivers or school staff in the diabetes management. The ADA has set out recommendations on how schools and day care centers should respond (see Resources) and how to set up a Diabetes Health Care Plan for your child.

In addition to providing all the supplies (insulin and syringes, log book, glucose meter, testing strips, glucagon injection, ketone testing strips, and glucose tablets or gel) for caring for your child's diabetes, you should also provide the following information to the caregivers at your child's day care or school:

- How and when your child's blood glucose should be monitored
- How to store the insulin and other supplies, such as testing strips, glucagon injection, and glucose tablets and gels
- When your child should eat (meal and snack schedule) and how much insulin should be given before these meals; if there are parties and special events at school, provide instructions on how much extra insulin should be given
- How your child behaves or what symptoms may indicate he or she is hypoglycemic, and how much glucose should be given when his or her blood glucose is low
- When and how to administer glucagon injection

- How your child behaves when the blood glucose is high and when and how to test for ketones
- Whom to contact in an emergency: parent and family phone numbers, doctor's phone numbers, and emergency room phone numbers

Children—Ages Eight to Eleven

At this age, children frequently do their own blood glucose testing and insulin injections. Many may use insulin pumps for the first time. You will still be involved in supervising at this stage—there is evidence that children do better if parents are involved. Children who develop diabetes at this age are more likely to get depressed and anxious, especially when the honeymoon phase ends and the child realizes that the diabetes is not going to go away and may get harder to manage. With parental encouragement and support, the child should participate in school activities and sports.

Adolescence

Adolescence, when there are physical changes of puberty as well as cognitive and emotional changes, brings some new challenges to managing diabetes.

- **Early adolescence—ages twelve to fifteen:** Puberty increases the insulin needs, so your child's medical team will make adjustments of the insulin dose. At this age, the child will do his or her own blood glucose monitoring and injections. You may need to negotiate with your child as to how much supervision is appropriate. It is a good idea to talk to your child about issues such as weight and body image. Occasionally an adolescent child

---

DID YOU KNOW?

Public Schools and Diabetes Training

In the United States, the schools or day care centers that receive public funds are legally required to provide training to school staff on treating diabetes. The ADA has literature for teachers and child-care providers. Your health-care team can also help ensure that the staff members at your child's school are adequately trained. The degree of supervision by the staff of the school will vary with your child's age and abilities.

may limit insulin use in order to lose weight. This leads to poor diabetes control and is harmful.

• **Late adolescence—ages fifteen to nineteen:** At this age your child will manage his or her diabetes fairly independently. You can help by guiding your teen to improve his or her coping skills and transition to full independence for college or work.

Diabetes can impact the adolescent issues of smoking, alcohol, risky behaviors, and sexual activity. Smoking increases the risk for diabetes complications. Let your teenager know how alcohol causes hypoglycemia and what can be done to prevent it (see Chapter 7). Discuss driving safety with your teenager, and let him or her know how important it is to check for hypoglycemia before and during driving. She also needs to know how diabetes can impact pregnancy and the importance of pregnancy planning. She can use oral contraception without medical risk. Both teenage sons and daughters need information about barrier contraception and prevention of sexually transmitted diseases.

With diabetes intruding into the teenager's struggle to separate from parents and the need to be accepted by peers, depression can occur, and if your child shows any signs of depression, he or she should get professional help.

GLUCOSE TARGETS FOR CHILDREN AND TEENAGERS

The targets for glucose control are different in early childhood because of the risks of hypoglycemia, and these targets need to be tailored for each child. Table 14-1 summarizes the ADA recommended goals for glucose levels in the different age groups.

Table 14-1 ADA Recommended Goals for Glucose Levels in Children and Adolescents			
Age	**Premeal Blood Glucose (mg/dl)**	**Bedtime and Middle of Night Blood Glucose (mg/dl)**	**HbA1c (Normal Is Less than 6)**
Under 6 years	100 to 180	110 to 200	7.5 to 8.5
6 to 11 years	90 to 160	100 to 180	Less than 8
12 to 19 years	90 to 130	90 to 150	Less than 7.5

Source: Silverstein J, Klingensmith G, Copeland K, Plotnick L, Kaufman F, Laffel L, Deeb L, Grey M, Anderson B, Holzmeister LA, Clark N, American Diabetes Association. "Care of children and adolescents with type 1 diabetes." *Diabetes Care* 2005; 28: 186–212.

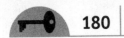

INSULIN THERAPY FOR CHILDREN

Adjusting Insulin Doses

Insulin dosages are based on weight of your child in kilograms (1 kg is equal to 2.2 pounds). The doses vary based on whether the child is in the honeymoon phase or not and whether he or she is going through puberty.

- During the honeymoon phase, your child will need very little insulin, and a simple insulin regimen with two or three injections a day may suffice. The basal insulin needs may be as low as 0.125 units per kilogram. The ratio for carbohydrate might be 1 unit of insulin for 60 to 75 grams carbohydrate, and your child may not need any insulin for corrections.

- Once the honeymoon phase is over, your child's basal insulin needs may go up to 0.25 units per kilogram, and the insulin to carbohydrate ratio may go up to 1 unit for 15 to 60 grams carbohydrate. He or she may also need insulin for correction, for example, 1 unit for every 50 to 200 mg/dl blood glucose over her target.

- When your child goes through puberty, the insulin needs go up substantially—this is principally because of the growth hormone pulses. Now the basal insulin requirements might be as much as 0.5 to 0.75 units per kilogram, the ratio for carbohydrate might be 1 unit for 8 to 10 grams carbohydrate, and the corrections for high sugars might be about 1 unit for 30 mg/dl blood glucose over target. Let your child know that this increase in dose is normal.

The dose ranges I have quoted are general guidelines; every child is different, and the doses your child's doctor will prescribe will depend on his or her age and size.

Working with Small Insulin Doses

Giving the small doses of insulin can be challenging. Eli Lilly and Novo Nordisk make pens that will deliver in half units, but the minimum dose is 1 unit. Becton, Dickinson and Company makes an ultrafine short-needle insulin syringe with half-unit markings. You can also ask your pharmacy to dilute the insulin. Eli Lilly makes a diluent for NPH, regular, and Humalog insulin. Similarly, Novo Nordisk makes a diluent for Novolin regular, and this can also be used for NovoLog. For U50 insulin, the insulin is diluted by 50 percent, so 1 ml contains 50 units of insulin. If you draw up 1 unit on an insulin syringe, you are giving 0.5 units. For U10 insulin, the insulin is diluted by 90 percent, so 1 ml contains 10 units of insulin. If you draw up 1 unit on an insulin syringe, you are giving 0.1 units.

The diluted insulin does not last as long, and you may need a new diluted batch every two weeks. If you use diluted insulin for your child, it is very important that all caregivers are aware of this to avoid giving the same amount of undiluted insulin.

Managing the Decreased Duration of the Action of Injected Insulin

Very young children need tiny amounts of insulin, and because the volumes of insulin are so small, the insulins work for shorter periods. Thus insulin glargine does not last for twenty-four hours and usually has to be given twice a day for basal coverage.

Injection Sites

Inject the insulin in the abdomen (avoid the two-inch area in the center—one inch either side of the umbilicus). Alternative places to inject include the front and side of thighs (top and outside is best), buttocks, and side of arms. Do not inject in the same spot again and again because it can cause lipohypertrophy, a thickening of the tissues that interferes with the absorption of insulin. After injecting with a pen, count to ten before removing the needle to avoid insulin leakage.

Limiting the Number of Injections

Children have multiple meals and snacks throughout the day, but insulin is not usually given for all the meals (this is especially true for babies). Usually, a basal insulin is given and then corrections made by giving extra doses as needed. If a child is unwilling to get an insulin injection at lunchtime at school, then a mixture of fast-acting insulin analog with NPH injected in the morning will cover breakfast and the lunchtime meal, provided the child is willing to eat a consistent amount of carbohydrate at lunch. The next injection can be fast-acting insulin with the after-school snack and/or dinner, and then an NPH injection at bedtime.

If your child needs her insulins to be mixed, use the following guidelines for mixing insulins:

- Draw up regular insulin or the fast-acting insulin analog first—then draw up the NPH (that is, "clear insulin before cloudy"). To prevent the formation of a vacuum in the vial, you are supposed to put an equal amount of air into the vial as the amount of insulin you are going to draw up. So, if you are going to draw up 3 units of Lispro and 7 units of NPH, you first put 7 units of air in the NPH bottle and then put 3 units of air in the Lispro bottle; next draw up 3 units of Lispro and then 7 units of NPH. You do not have to put air into vials if you use only a small amount of insulin in a vial every month before discarding it and opening a new vial.

• Even though mixing insulin glargine with the fast-acting insulin analogs is not recommended, you can do this provided it is done immediately before injecting—draw up the fast-acting insulin (lispro or insulin aspart) and then draw up the insulin glargine. The mixture does go cloudy, but go ahead and inject it anyway.

• Do not mix insulin detemir with insulin aspart: this reduces the effect of insulin aspart by 40 percent.

Using Small Needles

Use short needles for children because they do not have much fat. Inject at an angle to avoid giving intramuscular insulin, which would get absorbed much faster.

Handling a Fear of Needles

If your child has a fear of seeing the needle going into his or her skin during the injection, you can use a device called Inject-Ease, which hides the insulin syringe and needle. You place the device tip on the skin and press a button to give an injection (see Resources). There are also covers available that hide the needles within the pens—examples include the NovoPen 3 PenMate and NeedleAid.

Using Insulin Pumps

Insulin pumps are an increasingly popular alternative to injections in children (see Chapter 6). The main disadvantage of pumps is that if the infusion set gets kinked or dislodged or there is a pump malfunction, the child can go into ketoacidosis within a few hours. Pumps are great for children and families who are proactive in managing the diabetes.

IDENTIFICATION

Your child should wear her identification bracelet or necklace that alerts other people about her diabetes so that she can be appropriately treated if she loses consciousness. There are trendy ones that might appeal to adolescents and teens. For toddlers, shoe tags are available (see Resources). Wearing a diabetes ID is particularly important when adolescents start driving and spending more time away from home.

WHEN YOUR CHILD GETS SICK

Children with diabetes do not get more illnesses than children without diabetes. They may get the usual viral illness in the winter—colds and coughs, sometimes vomiting and diarrhea. When you are looking after your sick child, consider the following guidelines:

- Do not stop the insulin—depending on the severity of the illness, the child may need the same or more insulin. Illness raises stress hormones, and so more insulin than usual might be needed.

- Check your child's glucose levels more often—every two to four hours.

- Encourage your child to drink plenty of fluids—sips of water, diet soda, sugar-free lemonade, sugar-free Popsicles, and broth are all fine.

- Encourage your child to eat his usual meals, but if he won't, give him regular sodas, juice, Jell-O, or Gatorade.

- Check ketones—either in the urine or in the blood.

- It is all right to give your child over-the-counter cough medicines: don't worry about the sugar in these medicines.

- Cover the carbohydrates with insulin in the usual way (sometimes given after the food just to make sure that your child will keep the food or drink down). If the glucose is high, give additional insulin to correct this. If your child is on basal and bolus insulin or on a pump, the basal insulin should be kept going.

- You should have your glucagon handy just in case you gave additional insulin and your child then can't keep down carbohydrates and her glucose level is going low. Make up the glucagon by injecting all of the solution in the syringe into the vial of glucagon. Then use an insulin syringe to draw up and give the glucagon. Table 14-2 lists recommendations on how much glucagon to give.

Contact your child's medical team and go to the emergency room if

- She is vomiting or has diarrhea and is unable to keep down fluids

- Blood glucose levels remain high (more than 250 mg/dl) despite taking extra insulin

Table 14-2 How Much Glucagon to Give		
Age	Markings on Insulin Syringe	Micrograms of Glucagon
2 years old or younger	2-unit mark*	20
Older than 2 years	1 unit mark per year of age up to maximum of 15 unit marks*	20 to maximum of 150

*If the initial dose does not increase glucose after 30 minutes, you can give another injection at double the dose—that is, 4 unit markings for children younger than 2 years and 2 unit markings per year up to a maximum of 30 unit markings for children older than 2 years.

Source: Haymond MW, Schreiner B. "Mini-dose glucagon rescue for hypoglycemia in children with type 1 diabetes." *Diabetes Care* 2001; 24: 643–45.

- There are high levels of ketones in blood or urine
- She experiences abdominal pain, shortness of breath, or drowsiness

Throughout the year, keep your child's immunizations up to date. Your child and family members should also get the flu injection each year. Also be sure to review these sick day guidelines with your child's medical team on a periodic basis.

TESTING FOR AUTOIMMUNE DISEASES

I mentioned in Chapter 3 that people with type 1 diabetes are at risk for other autoimmune diseases, especially thyroid disease and celiac disease.

When your child is diagnosed with type 1 diabetes, he should also be screened for autoimmune thyroid disease. His doctor will do these thyroid tests at intervals or if there is a problem with your child's growth, because low thyroid hormone levels can slow down growth.

In celiac disease, eating foods containing gluten (that is, those derived from wheat, oats, rye, and barley) cause an autoimmune damage to the wall of the small bowel. This damage leads to diarrhea, abdominal pain, tiredness, problems absorbing vitamins such as vitamin B_{12}, poor weight gain, and decreased growth. It can also affect the absorption of carbohydrates, causing hypoglycemia. The treatment is a gluten-free diet. Screening for celiac disease is done when a diagnosis of type 1 diabetes is made, and then again if the child has problems such as growth failure or weight loss or gastrointestinal problems. The blood test that is done is called tissue transglutaminase IgA autoantibody. If the blood test is positive, then your child will need to see a gastroenterologist, who may do a small bowel biopsy to confirm the diagnosis. You need to be sure of the diagnosis because you do not want to put your child on a gluten-free diet unless it is absolutely necessary. A gluten-free diet should only be started after the diagnosis has been confirmed—starting it earlier may affect the results of the tests.

Type 2 Diabetes in Children

The number of children that have type 2 diabetes is on the rise. Accurate numbers about how many children have this condition are hard to obtain, because the disease may have been present for a while before it is diagnosed. Anywhere between 8 to 46 percent of children with diabetes referred to pediatric centers have type 2 diabetes. The increase in childhood obesity is likely to be the main factor driving this increased incidence of type 2 diabetes.

Your child might be diagnosed with diabetes during routine screening or because she may be unwell. The American Diabetes Association recommends screening any overweight child (more than 120 percent ideal body weight, body mass index greater than 85 percent) who has two of the following features:

- Strong family history of type 2 diabetes (parents, siblings, uncles, aunts, grandparents, nephew, niece, half sibling)

- High-risk ethnic background: African-American, Hispanic, American Indian, Asian, Pacific Islander

- Evidence for insulin resistance or presence of conditions associated with insulin resistance, such as darkening of the skin under the armpits or around the neck (acanthosis nigricans), high blood pressure, high triglyceride levels, or polycystic ovarian syndrome

The screening starts at age ten or at puberty, whichever is earlier, and is done every two years.

High glucose levels may lead to yeast or bladder infections. Occasionally, the child may present in hyperosmolar coma or even diabetic ketoacidosis (see Chapter 3). Also keep in mind that, in children, it is sometimes difficult to distinguish between type 1 and type 2 diabetes.

TREATMENT FOR TYPE 2 DIABETES IN CHILDREN

The treatment options for children with type 2 diabetes are the same as those available for adults with type 2 diabetes. They include diet, exercise, and oral and injectable medications including insulin. The problem with medications is that there is limited information about their long-term use in children.

Diet and exercise are central to treatment. Other family members are also likely to have a problem with weight, and therefore all family members will benefit if they participate in the diet and exercise plan.

Diet

Work with the nutritionist to create a healthy meal plan. Keep low-fat, low-calorie choices in the house—switch to leaner cuts of meat, poultry, and fish, lower-fat cheeses, and nonfat milk. Add more vegetables and fiber to the diet, and use fruits as desserts rather than cake, pie, cookies, and ice cream. Watch the size of each serving, and avoid second helpings. If weight loss is the goal, set reasonable weight-loss targets (usually no more than one-half to one pound of lost weight per week), and monitor your child's progress. Give your child rewards for achieving the goals.

Exercise

You can increase your child's physical activity by

- Limiting screen time (television, computer, and game consoles)
- Being a role model for your child by limiting your sedentary time
- Engaging your child in physical activities he or she enjoys—go for walks, enroll in team sports, play hoops in the back yard, or join a martial arts academy

The child should get a minimum of thirty to sixty minutes of physical exercise daily—and yes, that's every day! If your child is on sulfonylureas or insulin, hypoglycemia can occur with exercise. See Chapter 9 for safe exercise guidelines.

Medications

Metformin is approved for children and is the first medication to use. In addition to lowering glucose, it also helps with weight loss and also lowers triglyceride levels. For some children, the gastrointestinal symptoms may be a problem. If metformin alone is insufficient at controlling the blood glucose levels, sulfonylureas can be tried. There is a risk of hypoglycemia with the sulfonylureas, and some weight gain. The thiazolidinediones are being tested in children, but their main disadvantage in children (and adults) is that they do cause weight gain. Also, in adults, the thiazolidinediones have been implicated in bone loss, and rosiglitazone may increase the risk of heart attacks. Exenatide causes weight loss, but there is no information on its use in children.

For children whose diabetes is not controlled with metformin and sulfonylurea, insulin should be considered. The child usually stays on the oral medications and insulin is added. Initially you can just add a bedtime dose of insulin glargine or detemir and adjust the dose to get fasting glucose to goal. If the premeal glucose levels go up, add a fast-acting insulin analog before meals. If the child is reluctant to take multiple injections, premixed 75/25 Humalog mix or 70/30 NovoLog mix twice a day can be tried.

A number of children with type 2 diabetes actually have significant insulin deficiency, which explains why they got diabetes so early in life and why insulin may be the right treatment.

The doses of insulin in children with type 2 diabetes are usually higher than in children with type 1 diabetes because of the insulin resistance. However, your child's doctor may start him off at doses similar to those used for children with type 1 diabetes and then increase the doses as needed, based on his glucose levels.

Blood Pressure

It is particularly important to measure a child's blood pressure if there is a family history of high blood pressure. Children's blood pressures vary depending on age, sex, and height. If the blood pressure is high on repeated measurements, the pediatrician may do further investigations (including blood tests and looking at the kidney blood vessels using ultrasound). If there is no other abnormality that is responsible for the elevated blood pressure, then the child is treated. A reduced-calorie diet, more exercise, and a no-added-salt diet may help. If this treatment is not sufficient, the child may be prescribed an ACE inhibitor or additional blood pressure medications as necessary (see Chapter 3).

Lipid Profile

Children who are older than two years should have a lipid profile done at diagnosis of diabetes if they have a family history of coronary artery disease or if the family history is unknown. If there is no family history of coronary artery disease, then the lipid profile should be done at puberty. Children should have an LDL cholesterol less than 100 mg/dl. Treatment is principally with diet, although statin medications are recommended for LDL cholesterol over 160 mg/dl. Ezetimibe has also been approved for use in children over ten years of age. If the lipids are normal, they should be checked again every five years.

SCREENING FOR COMPLICATIONS

Annual screening for microalbuminuria (see Chapter 5) starts once the child is ten years old and has had diabetes for five years.

Diabetic eye disease (retinopathy) is more common after puberty but can occur earlier. The first exam should occur once the child is ten years old and has had diabetes for three to five years.

Foot problems are rare in children. Still, your child should get a foot examination yearly starting at puberty.

See Chapters 3 and 5 for information on screening for complications. Many of the same rules that apply for adult screening apply for children as well.

Summary

- The younger your child, the more involved you will to be in the day-to-day management of the diabetes.

- When the child goes to school, you will need to involve the school in the diabetes management.

- The adolescent child is increasingly able to take on the day-to-day management of his or her diabetes, but you should still stay involved.

- Hypoglycemia is of major concern in young children, and the glucose targets are higher than in adults.

- Make sure you know how to deal with the diabetes when your child is sick:

  - Continue to give the insulin.

  - Monitor blood glucose levels frequently.

  - In case of persistent hypoglycemia, make sure that you know how to use minidose glucagon.

- Children with type 1 diabetes are at increased risk for other autoimmune diseases, and your child will be screened for celiac disease and autoimmune thyroid disease.

- The number of children with type 2 diabetes is increasing. The treatment options for children with type 2 diabetes include diet, exercise, and oral and injectable medications including insulin.

- There is limited information about the long-term use of oral diabetes medications in children. Metformin is approved for children. If metformin alone is insufficient, sulfonylureas can be added. If these two drugs are insufficient, then insulin is added.

Diabetes Camps

I encourage children with diabetes and their families to attend diabetes camp. For a week or two, it is great for the child and his or her family to live among people for whom checking glucose and adjusting insulin doses is the norm rather than the exception. Your child can learn about the latest techniques in diabetes management. Parents can get some relief from the daily task of being diabetes manager. Adolescent camps and college preparation camps can help with the transition from close parental involvement to the independence of the young adult. The ADA and Children with Diabetes websites have information about diabetes camps (see Resources).

CHAPTER 15

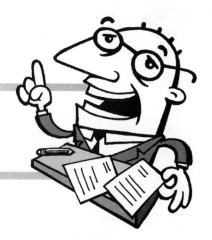

Diabetes as You Age

The likelihood of developing diabetes increases as you get older. Almost 20 percent of people older than sixty-five have diabetes, and this number increases to almost 40 percent of people over age eighty. This is partly because people with diabetes are living longer and also because aging is associated with decreases in insulin secretion from the pancreas. With people living longer, diabetes is therefore a major health issue in old age. The majority of elderly people with diabetes have type 2 diabetes, but type 1 diabetes can also occur.

There are a number of issues that need to be considered when discussing diabetes in the elderly population:

- Blood glucose targets
- How physical changes that occur with aging will affect diabetes management
- How diabetes will impact other diseases of aging
- Treatment of diabetes complications and associated disorders (for example, blood pressure and lipid levels)
- How drug interactions will affect the treatment of diabetes and other diseases

Blood Glucose Targets in the Elderly

When you think about glucose targets in elderly people with diabetes, it is helpful to separate those elderly people who developed diabetes when they were younger from people who develop the disease in old age.

If you were young when you developed diabetes, you have already established targets for glucose control, and it may not be necessary to change them as you age. However, if you have complications from diabetes, your targets may need to be changed to reflect your current disease state.

What about blood glucose targets in elderly people who have been newly diagnosed with diabetes? When setting blood glucose targets for elderly people, doctors take into consideration the life expectancy of the individual, because this will affect how the diabetes is managed.

The average life expectancy for a sixty-five-year-old woman in the United States is nineteen years, and for a man, it is fifteen years. At age seventy-five, the life expectancy is twelve and nine years respectively. Thus, after age seventy-five, what matters more is glycemic control to prevent short-term complications and not necessarily long-term complications. This is illustrated in Table 15-1, which examines the relationship between HbA1c and the lifetime risk of blindness, depending on the age at which you develop diabetes. So, if you are forty-five and had poor glucose control, your lifetime risk of becoming blind is high (7.9 percent), whereas if you are seventy-five and had the same glucose level, your likelihood of going blind due to diabetes is only 0.5 percent. In other words, there is a change in the risk-benefit analysis equation.

Even though there may be less concern about long-term complications, good glucose control is still important to prevent infections such as urinary tract infections and yeast infections. Glucose control will also impact your general nutritional state

Table 15-1	HbA1c and the Lifetime Risk of Blindness (in %)		
HbA1c	**Diabetes Develops at Age 45**	**Diabetes Develops at Age 65**	**Diabetes Develops at Age 75**
7	0.3	<0.1	<0.1
8	1.1	0.2	<0.1
9	2.6	0.5	0.1
10	5.0	1.0	0.3
11	7.9	1.9	0.5

Source: Adapted from Vijan S, Hofer TP, Hayward RA. "Estimated benefits of glycemic control in microvascular complications in type 2 diabetes." *Ann Intern Med* 1997 Nov 1; 127 (9): 788–95.

and your sense of well-being. The American Geriatrics Society recommends an HbA1c goal of less than 8 percent in frail individuals (frail meaning people who do not have much physical reserve and become ill easily) with a life expectancy of less than five years, or when risks of intensive glycemic control outweigh benefits. For healthy people over seventy-five, the HbA1c target of less than 7 percent is the same as in younger individuals. Your age, your health status, and your motivation to control your diabetes are all taken into account when your doctor is setting blood glucose targets for you.

How Aging Affects Diabetes Management

The following sections discuss how the physical changes that occur as the body ages will affect the management of diabetes.

METABOLISM OF MEDICATIONS

As you get older, your kidney function declines, so the effects of many oral diabetes medications and insulin last longer. Therefore, your doctor will avoid (or use more cautiously) the long-acting sulfonylureas such as glyburide and glimepiride that are more likely to result in low glucose reactions. Instead, he or she will use the fast-acting sulfonylureas (glipizide or tolbutamide), or nateglinide or repaglinide. However, this makes more frequent dosing necessary, and this may make it harder to remember to take your medications. Kidney function can also decline when an elderly person is ill and becomes dehydrated (for example with pneumonia). If this happens and the person is taking metformin for diabetes, the amount of metformin in the bloodstream can go up and cause a serious condition called lactic acidosis. For this reason your doctor will most likely prescribe lower doses of metformin and do blood tests to monitor your kidney function, especially when you are ill.

HEART DISEASE

Elderly patients are more likely to have had a heart attack or have heart disease due to high blood pressure. They are more prone to develop heart failure, and so doctors will avoid (or use cautiously) medicines such as rosiglitazone or pioglitazone that can precipitate heart failure.

If an older patient has angina, hypoglycemia is more dangerous because it can precipitate an angina attack. Therefore, doctors are cautious in using insulin and oral medications that cause hypoglycemia in people with angina.

MALNOURISHMENT

When an elderly person is acutely ill, the loss of appetite can deplete the liver glycogen stores, and this increases the risk of hypoglycemia, especially at night. If an elderly person has dementia or has had a stroke, swallowing can become impaired, and this too can increase the risk of hypoglycemia. Under these circumstances, the diabetes medicines tolbutamide, nateglinide, and repaglinide can be given before each meal, and if the person is not eating, the dose can be skipped.

NEUROLOGICAL CHANGES

Elderly people may not have as many symptoms in response to hypoglycemia (tremor, sweating, fast heart rate, hunger), and so they may not recognize low glucose reactions as well as younger individuals do. This can cause a delay in treatment, and glucose levels can go dangerously low. If an elderly person is delirious because of an acute illness or is chronically confused because of dementia, his or her caregivers may have difficulty recognizing and treating low glucose reactions.

The perception of thirst is often altered in older people, and if they do not drink enough, they can become dehydrated and have elevated glucose levels. This is especially a problem when the person is immobile and does not have ready access to water.

Memory changes in the elderly can impact their ability to manage diabetes. For example, they may not remember to take the medications. They may not be able to draw up or adjust the insulin doses for the food eaten. When this happens, caregivers may need to remind them to take their medications and supervise the insulin injections.

MOBILITY

Elderly people who have difficulty walking may have problems getting to the kitchen to treat their low glucose levels, so they should keep fast-acting carbohydrates such as glucose tablets close by.

Exercise remains important in elderly people with diabetes—it may reduce the person's need for additional medicines to control the glucose levels, and he or she is less likely to fall down.

VISION

As a person ages, his or her vision may deteriorate because of cataracts or macular disease, and it may be harder to monitor glucose levels. Using a magnifying glass when drawing up insulin, or better still, using insulin pens to dose the insulin, may make things easier.

ARTHRITIS

Osteoarthritis and rheumatoid arthritis of the hands can make it harder to open bottles of medicines, to draw up insulin, or to use pens. Novo Nordisk makes a disposable, prefilled Novolin InnoLet insulin doser, which has a large, easy-to-read dial, with audible clicks, to make it easier to select and inject the correct dose of insulin.

How Diabetes Impacts Diseases of Aging

Elderly people with long-standing diabetes are more likely to have kidney disease, nerve damage, and circulation problems such as heart disease and stroke. They are less able to walk, do housework, prepare meals, and manage money when compared to age-matched individuals who do not have diabetes. Women with diabetes become disabled at approximately twice the rate of women without diabetes, and they have an increased risk of falls and hip fractures. Long-standing diabetes can affect bone quality, and diabetes increases the risk of fractures with falls.

Neurological deterioration is greater in people with diabetes: they are more likely to develop memory problems and have more rapid deterioration in memory with time. Part of the reason for the more severe deterioration in cognitive function may be the effect of diabetes on the blood vessels and increased risk of small strokes.

Institutional Aspects of Diabetes

Elderly people living in board and care and nursing facilities may have additional challenges regarding their diabetes management. They may have to rely on caregivers to check their glucose levels and administer their diabetes medications. They may not have control over their meals. The staff may have limited understanding of diabetes management—because type 2 diabetes is so much more common, people tend not to remember that older individuals can have type 1 diabetes. These type 1 patients may not get adequate insulin bolus for their meals. Due to limited supervision, sophisticated insulin basal-bolus regimens may not be realistic, and some level of control may have to be sacrificed for safety. In these situations, insulin injections once or twice a day may have to suffice.

I would encourage family members to remain actively engaged in helping manage their elderly relative's diabetes care, and with their physician, carefully devise recommendations for the nursing staff in the residential home.

Treatment of Diabetes Complications and Associated Disorders

Diabetes complications in elderly people are treated in the same ways as in younger individuals. Treating the lipid abnormalities (see Chapter 3) and blood pressure is equally beneficial in the elderly as in younger individuals. In fact, because the risk for heart attack and stroke is higher in the elderly, benefits may actually be greater than in the younger population. The blood pressure target is less than 140/80 if tolerated. ACE inhibitors and angiotensin receptor blockers (ARBs) can be used to lower blood pressure, but these medicines can raise the potassium and serum creatinine levels. High potassium levels can be dangerous and affect the heart rhythm. Therefore, your doctor will ask you to get lab tests one week after you start taking these medicines to make sure that your potassium is in the safe range.

Often, elderly people are on many different medications because they are being treated for other medical problems as well. In these situations, you need to watch out for drug interactions between medications, because they will affect your well-being. For example, if you are taking glipizide for your diabetes, taking an antibiotic called ciprofloxacin can sometimes cause low glucose reactions.

Prednisone, a steroid that is given for bronchitis and rheumatological conditions such as acute gout, polymyalgia rheumatica, and other inflammatory conditions, can cause glucose levels to go high, and adjustments in your diabetes medications may be necessary.

If you are taking nitrate medicines for heart disease, you cannot use the phosphodiesterase inhibitors (sildenafil, vardenafil, or tadalafil) for erectile dysfunction.

So, when you get a new medicine prescription from your doctor, talk to your pharmacist and make sure that the new medicine will not interact with the medications you are already taking.

Summary

- Diabetes is more likely to occur as you age.
- The blood glucose targets are the same as in younger individuals except in frail individuals, when an HbA1c level of less than 8 percent is acceptable.
- The treatment options are the same as in younger individuals except that you need to take into account the changes related to aging (such as vision,

dexterity, mobility, and memory) and other medical problems (such as heart and kidney failure).

- Diabetes self-management is important—work with your medical team (the nutritionist, diabetes educator, and primary care physician or endocrinologist) to design the treatment plan appropriate for you.

- If you or your family member with diabetes is living in a residential home, work with the medical team and caregivers at the home to make sure that everybody knows how the diabetes should be managed.

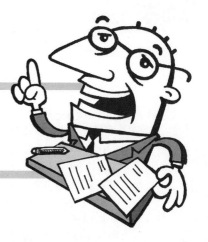

CHAPTER 16

Putting It All Together

This chapter integrates all the information in this book on how to manage type 1 and type 2 diabetes.

Type 1 Diabetes

Managing type 1 diabetes requires diligence, practice, and patience, as well as a good support team.

NEWLY DIAGNOSED TYPE 1 DIABETES

When you are first diagnosed with type 1 diabetes, you will meet your diabetes management team, which consists of your physician, the diabetes educator, and the nutritionist.

The physician will answer your questions about diabetes and recommend an initial insulin regimen. The nutritionist will teach you about carbohydrate counting, give you a carbohydrate exchange book (the ADA publishes a good one), and explain how to read food labels. She will also describe how to have a balanced diet and tell you about the best sources of fast-acting carbohydrates that can be used to treat low glucose levels.

The diabetes educator will teach you how to use a glucose monitor, how to keep a logbook, and how often you should monitor your glucose levels and will set your target glucose levels. She will also teach you how to draw up insulin in a syringe and give an injection. Even if you were prescribed insulin pens from the start, you should still know how to draw up insulin in a syringe just in case a pen is not available. The educator will go over the symptoms of low glucose reactions and how to treat them. She will also show you how glucagon works and instruct you and a family member on its use. She will give you information about the resources available in your community for people with diabetes. She will explain how you can incorporate taking care of your diabetes into your day-to-day activities and how to involve family, friends, and colleagues.

Usually, newly diagnosed people with type 1 diabetes still make insulin, and initially, low doses of insulin are required and glucose control is relatively easy. This is called the honeymoon phase. During this period, the glucose levels go up with meals only, so you can start treatment with an insulin pen of a fast-acting insulin analog before each meal using insulin pens that allow you to inject half-unit doses of insulin. The initial ratio might be 1 unit of insulin for 30 to 45 grams carbohydrate. If your glucose is high, you may need additional insulin to bring down the number—this is called correction insulin. The ratio for correction might be 1 unit of insulin for every 75 mg/dl blood glucose over a target of 150. For example, if your premeal blood glucose was 225 and you were going to eat 30 grams carbohydrate, you would inject 1 unit of insulin for correction plus 1 unit for carbohydrates, or a total of 2 units fast-acting insulin analog.

Initially, your medical team will see you quite frequently (at one- to two-week intervals) to review the glucose levels and help you with insulin adjustments. If possible, you should also attend a course on diabetes self-management, with the goal of understanding all aspects of diabetes management.

ESTABLISHED TYPE 1 DIABETES

Currently, there is no way of preventing the decline in insulin secretion that occurs with time in those with type 1 diabetes. The honeymoon period can last only a few weeks, or it can last for more than a year or two. Generally speaking, children and young adults tend to have shorter honeymoons, whereas older individuals can maintain insulin secretion for several years. There are, however, many exceptions to this observation.

As your insulin secretion declines, you will need more insulin to control the glucose. You may find that your glucose values drift upward overnight. This is a good time to add some long-acting basal insulin. Usually only a few units (2 to 3) of insulin glargine or detemir might be necessary to start with, but then the doses go up with time. The ratios of insulin for carbohydrate and for correction also change, and more insulin is needed. The amount of insulin that you need will vary according to your age and weight: a teenager going through puberty will need almost twice as much insulin as a man in his mid-thirties or older. Table 16-1 gives you an approximation of the amount of insulin needed at different ages.

As the honeymoon fades, not only do your insulin requirements increase, but there is increased lability in the glucose levels. Therefore, you have to measure glucose levels more frequently and do more insulin injections during this period, and you and your medical team may decide that it is advantageous for you to go on an insulin pump (see Chapter 6).

YOUR GLUCOSE TARGET

The targets for glucose levels are

- 90 to 130 mg/dl before meals
- Less than 180 mg/dl after meals
- 100 to 130 mg/dl at bedtime and at 2 A.M.

Table 16-1 Amount of Insulin Needed			
	Basal Units per Kilogram (1 kilogram = 2.2 pounds)	Ratio for Carbohydrates: Units of Insulin per Gram Carbohydrate	Ratio for Correction: Units of Insulin per mg/dl Glucose over Target Level (Usually 100 to 120)
Newly diagnosed (in honeymoon)	0.125	1/30 (0.5/15)*	1/100 (0.5/50)
Puberty (established)	0.35	1/8 to 1/10	1/25 to 1/40
Young adult (established)	0.25 to 0.3	1/10 to 1/12	1/40 to 1/50
Older adult (established)	0.25	1/15	1/50

*Another way of thinking about ratios is to keep the denominators unchanged at 15 for carbohydrates and 50 at correction and change the numerator. Thus if you give 0.5 units for 15 grams carbohydrate, the correction will be 0.5 units for 50 mg/dl glucose over target. If you give 1 unit for 15 grams carbohydrate, the correction will be 1 unit for 50 mg/dl glucose over target.

If you give enough insulin, everyone can reach these targets, but at the expense of lots of hypoglycemic reactions. The goal is to maximize the times you are in this range with as few hypoglycemic reactions as possible.

To reach these targets safely, you can do the following:

Optimizing Your Basal Insulin Dose

Ideally, if your basal insulin (insulin glargine, detemir, NPH, or pump basal) dose is correct, then even if you did not eat and had your normal activity, your glucose levels will stay in the normal range. This is usually not true in practice, and there is always some drift in your glucose levels. This is because of the day-to-day variability in the absorption of the injected insulin and the way the body responds to the insulin. Your goal is to minimize the upward and downward drift of your glucose levels.

So, how do you determine if your basal insulin dose is correct? You do this by looking at your glucose levels after eliminating the variables of food, exercise, and bolus insulin. Usually, overnight is the easiest time to assess your basal insulin needs:

- Eat early in the evening, and limit your carbohydrates so that by bedtime there is no effect of the evening bolus and your stomach is empty.

- Provided your glucose at bedtime is in the safe range—say 100 to 150 mg/dl, then you can set your alarm and check blood glucose levels at 2 A.M. and then again at 6 A.M. and 9 A.M. If your glucose levels drift up or down, you need more or less basal insulin respectively.

Once you have determined that your overnight basal is satisfactory, then you can work on determining the basal doses during the day. The principal is the same—you want to look for glucose drift after you eliminate the effect of food, bolus insulin, and exercise. Instead of fasting all day, try limited fasts:

- If you want to know that your morning basal dose is correct, then on a day when your fasting glucose is on target, do not eat breakfast or give bolus insulin, and instead plan to eat an early lunch. You can check glucose levels throughout the morning and look for glucose drift.

- If you are interested in determining whether the early afternoon basal doses are correct, eat breakfast but delay or skip lunch.

- If you are interested in late afternoon basal doses, then either have an early lunch with limited carbohydrates or skip lunch.

- If you are interested in early evening basal doses, delay dinner. An early dinner or skipping dinner will allow you to evaluate late evening basal doses.

You need to confirm your observations because of day-to-day variability. In other words, after checking glucose levels overnight, if you think that your glucose levels are drifting upward and that you need more basal insulin, check again (preferably twice) to make sure this is a consistent finding before making the intervention.

If you perform the above analysis you may find

- Your glucose levels are stable if you do eat or give bolus insulin—your once-daily dose of injectable basal insulin or pump basals are working just fine.

- Your glucose value drifts downward or upward overnight and you need to increase or decrease your basal insulin respectively.

- Your glucose levels are stable most of the night but shoot up at around 5 to 6 A.M. In other words you have a strong dawn phenomenon. If you are on an insulin pump, you can adjust the basal rate on your pump to cover this dawn phenomenon. If you are on a long-acting basal insulin injection you have several options:

  - Carefully increase your nighttime insulin to see if you can get away with it—the concern is that you might go low earlier in the night.

  - Change your basal insulin. For example, if you are on insulin glargine, you could try insulin detemir, which has more of a peak.

  - Wake up at 5 A.M. every day and give a little bolus insulin.

  - This is a good reason for switching from insulin injections to an insulin pump (see Chapter 6).

- Your glucose levels drift up midafternoon when you do not eat lunch or give a bolus. This tells you that your injected basal insulin is not lasting twenty-four hours or you need to increase the afternoon basal rate on your pump. If this occurs on long-acting basal injection, then I would recommend splitting your basal insulin and giving it twice a day. Usually you will need more in the evening to cover the dawn phenomenon and a smaller dose in the morning.

Once you have determined that your basal doses are reasonable and that any drift is minimized, you cannot assume that they will stay the same. They will change for a number of reasons:

- Change in activity is an obvious cause—often, people find that they have to increase their basal insulin during winter, when they are spending more time indoors.

- Stress can have an impact—some people find that they need more insulin when they are stressed.

- There can be changes relating to the menstrual cycle. Some, but not all, women find that they need more insulin in the second half of their cycle, especially the five days before their period. As soon as their period starts, they become more sensitive and have to cut back on their basal insulin. If you are on a pump, it is quite easy to use a different set of basals for different times of your cycle.

I do want to emphasize that assessing basal doses is a reiterative process—you should evaluate them on a regular basis.

Optimizing Your Bolus Insulin Dose

Once you are satisfied with your basal glucose control, you can look at the bolus insulin. Before you can do this, you have to know how to count carbohydrates (see Chapter 8).

The way you assess your bolus ratio for carbohydrates is to eat your usual meal and give the calculated dose of insulin. Then check your blood glucose after the meal and find out how high it goes—you are trying to keep it below 180 mg/dl. Check three times, and if the glucose goes much higher than 180 consistently, you need to increase the ratio. For example, if you gave 1 unit for 15 grams carbohydrate at breakfast, try using 1 unit per 12 grams of carbohydrate, and check again. Sometimes, if you change the ratio, you find that your peak after the meal is below 180 mg/dl, but then you go low later on. If this happens, you have a number of options:

- You can try giving your bolus a little earlier: say, fifteen minutes before eating, rather than immediately before eating.

- You might decide to have a snack to prevent the low glucose level.

- If you are on a pump, you could reduce your basal temporarily at the time when you predict you will go low.

- A newer solution to this problem is to use pramlintide (Symlin)—this drug is injected before the meal, and it lowers postmeal glucose levels by suppressing glucagon levels after the meal and by delaying stomach emptying. The starting dose is 2.5 units of pramlintide, and it is incrementally increased by 2.5 units every few days to a maximum of 10 units before each meal. Pramlintide can cause nausea, and some people can only tolerate lower doses. If you are prescribed pramlintide, you will need to back off on your meal bolus ratio. How much you back off is variable: you may need to change the bolus from 1 unit for 15 grams carbohydrate to 1 unit for 20 to 30 grams carbohydrate.

Why do you have a correction insulin bolus? The correction insulin is to correct the drift upward in your glucose levels because the basal insulin is not perfect. The other reason for having a correction insulin bolus is if you underestimated the effect of the carbohydrate in a meal, and so underdosed your meal insulin, causing the glucose levels to run high. To figure out your correction ratio, look at your insulin bolus for carbohydrates:

- If you need 1 unit of insulin for 15 grams carbohydrate, 1 unit will lower your blood glucose by 50 mg/dl.

- If you need 1.5 units of insulin for 15 grams carbohydrate (that is 1 per 10 grams carbohydrate), then 1.5 units will lower your blood glucose by 50 mg/dl—or 1 unit will lower your blood glucose by 33 mg/dl (50 ÷ 1.5 = 1 unit per 33 mg/dl).

Monitoring Blood Glucose Levels

The risk of hypoglycemia goes up as you aim for glucose levels close to normal, and you will need to check your blood glucose frequently. You may end up checking eight to twelve times a day—before each meal, midmorning, midafternoon, bedtime, before and after exercise, before driving, sometimes at 2 A.M., and anytime you have symptoms that suggest hypoglycemia. You cannot achieve a normal HbA1c value safely if you check your blood glucose levels only three or four times a day.

Record your glucose values, the amount of carbohydrate you eat, the bolus insulin doses, and any exercise in a logbook, and review the data each week. Try to look for patterns of glucose levels. The continuous glucose monitoring systems can also help with identifying particular patterns of glucose fluctuations (see Chapter 5).

Counting Carbohydrates

To control your diabetes, you need to give the correct dose of insulin for the carbohydrate content of a meal. It may be relatively easy to do this at home but can be difficult when you eat out, especially if you order foods with sweet sauces. If you eat out a lot, this can significantly impact your overall glucose control. There are several ways you can approach this problem:

- Cut back on eating out.
- Work with your nutritionist to get better at estimating the carbohydrate content of restaurant foods and obtain nutrition guides that list the carbohydrate content of fast foods and other foods you eat.

- Keep notes of foods you eat and what happens to your glucose levels when you eat them, and make adjustments the next time. It becomes easier if you tend to eat the same meal when you go to your favorite restaurant.

The more consistent you are with your diet and activity, the easier it is to control your glucose levels.

Being Proactive

Make changes to your insulin doses if you think it necessary. Usually you should make small changes and then check to make sure that the change is working and not causing hypoglycemia.

Incorporating Diabetes Management into Your Daily Routine

It is easy to make changes for short periods of time, but harder to sustain them. This is when the people in your support network can help (see Chapter 4).

Type 2 Diabetes

In this section, I integrate information in this book about how to manage type 2 diabetes.

PREDIABETES

If you have a strong family history of diabetes, affecting your parents and siblings, then you are at risk for developing diabetes. Your physician can check your fasting glucose or do a two-hour glucose tolerance test (see Chapter 1) and tell you if you have either impaired fasting glucose (IFG) or impaired glucose tolerance (IGT). If you have these conditions or if you had diabetes during pregnancy (gestational diabetes), then you have **prediabetes** and are at risk for developing diabetes in the future. You are also at risk for developing heart disease.

If you have prediabetes, the recommended treatment is diet and exercise—losing 5 percent of your total body weight if you are overweight or obese will significantly delay the development of diabetes. If you are unable to lose weight or exercise, then medications are another option. In research studies, metformin, thiazolidinediones (rosiglitazone and pioglitazone), and acarbose have been shown to reduce the number of patients that progress to diabetes. At this time, however, none of these medications have been approved for use in diabetes prevention.

The increased risk for heart disease in people with prediabetes means that you should also get treated for high blood pressure and you should aim to get your LDL cholesterol below 100 mg/dl, using medications if necessary.

GETTING DIAGNOSED

People may be diagnosed with type 2 diabetes in a number of different ways:

- On routine blood tests
- Due to symptoms of high glucose levels—thirst, blurred vision, and weight loss
- Sometimes the glucose levels are so high that the patient may have severe dehydration and confusion or coma (hyperosmolar coma)
- Infections—bladder, vaginal, or penile yeast infection may indicate diabetes
- Long-term complications of diabetes—such as a foot ulcer—may also indicate diabetes

TREATING TYPE 2 DIABETES

Once your diabetes is diagnosed, your treatment will depend on how it was discovered. The therapies may include diet and exercise, oral medications, injectable non-insulin therapies, and insulin.

Education

After diagnosis, you will meet with a diabetes educator and a nutritionist. The diabetes educator will

- Teach you how to monitor glucose levels and keep a blood glucose log, as well as how to inject insulin or exenatide if your doctor prescribes them.
- Explain symptoms and treatment of hypoglycemia if you are going to take medication that could cause low glucose reactions.

The nutritionist will

- Teach you about the carbohydrate content of food
- Discuss weight-reducing strategies if this is indicated (see Chapter 10)

In addition to individual instruction, you should attend an educational course geared toward patients with type 2 diabetes. Your diabetes care team should be able to give you information about courses in your area.

Diet and Exercise

If the diagnosis was made on a routine blood test and the glucose levels are in the 130 to 160 mg/dl range, and you are overweight, your doctor may initially recommend that you go on a diet and exercise regularly. You may be able to get your glucose levels in the target range if you stop drinking regular sodas and juices and lose a little bit of weight.

Medicines

If your glucose levels do not come into the target range with diet and exercise, then you will be given metformin therapy. Metformin lowers glucose levels, and it also helps with weight loss. In a large research study called the UKPDS, obese patients with type 2 diabetes who took metformin had less microvascular and macrovascular events (see Chapter 3). If you need additional therapy that normally causes weight gain (insulin or sulfonylureas), the weight gain is less if you are also taking metformin.

If your diagnosis is made because you were admitted to a hospital with dehydration and very high glucose levels (hyperosmolar coma), then you will most probably start off with insulin therapy. If you are doing well a few weeks later, your doctor will probably add metformin and gradually reduce the insulin doses. Often the insulin can be stopped and the glucose levels controlled with metformin and perhaps a sulfonylurea.

If your glucose level is 200 mg/dl at diagnosis, your doctor will immediately start you on metformin therapy in addition to the diet and exercise therapy. Usually you will take 500 mg of metformin once a day with either breakfast or dinner and then increase it to 500 mg twice a day. Taking metformin with food helps reduce the gastrointestinal discomfort that can occur with the drug. The dose is increased to 1,000 mg twice a day if the glucose levels are above target. Sometimes you may get diarrhea with metformin—if this happens to you, you can work with your doctor to see if you can cut back and take a lower dose.

If diet, exercise, and metformin are insufficient, your doctor may add a second medicine. Which one he or she prescribes depends on your specific needs:

- If your glucose levels are in the target range all the time except after dinner, when you tend to eat more, then a fast-acting insulin-stimulating drug like tolbutamide, repaglinide, or nateglinide before dinner may suffice. Nateglinide is also very safe in older patients.

- If you are prone to having an increase in glucose levels overnight (due to the liver making excessive glucose), your doctor may give you a low dose of glyburide or glimepiride or glipizide with the evening meal. These medicines might work well in combination with metformin for a number of years. The risks are hypoglycemia and weight gain.

- When combined with metformin, rosiglitazone or pioglitazone also work well and can get the glucose levels on target. The metformin ameliorates some of the weight gain that occurs with these drugs. Your doctor may consider this option if you have a fatty liver because there is evidence that rosiglitazone and pioglitazone can help this problem. These drugs can't be used if you have heart failure or if you have fluid retention. Almost everybody who responds to these drugs gains weight, and this can be upsetting. Also, because of recent concerns with rosiglitazone regarding increased risk of heart attack, pioglitazone is the preferred option.

- Exenatide has the advantage that it makes you lose weight. The disadvantages are that it has to be given by injection and long-term safety data is lacking. Nausea is a side effect of exenatide, and if you have gastroparesis, you will not be able to use this drug.

- When combined with metformin, sitagliptin lowers glucose levels without increasing the risk of hypoglycemia. A theoretical advantage for this medication is that it may prevent further beta cell loss, but so far this has not been shown in humans. You do not lose weight with sitagliptin. The main side effects appear to be a slight increase in the white cells in the blood and sore throat.

If two medications do not control the glucose levels and get the HbA1c to target, your doctor may add a third medication. The following combinations can be effective:

- Metformin plus thiazolidinedione plus exenatide

- Metformin plus exenatide plus sulfonylurea

- Metformin plus thiazolidinedione plus sulfonylurea

If three medications are not sufficient, you could take a fourth medication, but most likely your doctor will recommend adding insulin. Your doctor may consider insulin earlier if you have medical conditions that make use of the other medications difficult.

There are many ways of starting insulin. One simple approach is to add 8 to 10 units of insulin glargine to your other diabetes medicines and every three days increase the dose by 2 units until the fasting glucose levels are less than 130 mg/dl. A lot of times this one injection of insulin plus the other diabetes medications is sufficient to get the glucose levels close to the normal range. If the glucose levels do

Table 16-2 Medications for Type 2 Diabetes

	Sulfonylureas, Nateglinide, Repaglinide	Alpha-Glucosidase Inhibitors	Metformin	Thiazolidinediones (Rosiglitazone, Pioglitazone)	Exenatide (by injection)	Sitagliptin	Pramlintide (by injection)	Insulins
Conditions in which medication cannot be used		Kidney failure Liver failure	Kidney failure	Heart failure Liver failure	Gastroparesis		Gastroparesis	
Beneficial effects apart from lowering glucose			Weight loss Lowers triglycerides May prevent circulatory problems In combination therapy limits weight gain associated with other diabetes medications	Improves lipids May prevent reblockage after cardiac stents Improves fatty liver	Weight loss Reduces programmed beta cell death (apoptosis) in mice and cell culture	Reduces programmed beta cell death (apoptosis) in mice and cell culture	Weight loss	
Side effects	Hypoglycemia Weight gain	Gastro-intestinal problems	Gastro-intestinal problems	Weight gain Fluid retention Heart failure May cause bone loss Rosiglitazone may increase risk of heart attack	Nausea Vomiting	Sore throat Increase in white blood cell count	Nausea Vomiting	Hypoglycemia Weight gain

drift up during the day, then a fast-acting insulin analog can be used before meals. At this point you should adjust the insulin for food in much the same way as a person with type 1 diabetes does (see Chapter 8 or the preceding section on type 1 diabetes).

Table 16-2 summarizes the available medications. Which medication you'll take depends on the glucose lowering effect and also what other benefits or risks the medication has. The benefits may be weight loss or triglyceride lowering, while the risks may be low glucose reactions, gastrointestinal symptoms, weight gain, and fluid retention.

Bariatric surgery is an option for people who are very heavy (BMI more than 35). You may be a candidate if you are having a difficult time controlling your glucose levels with the medicines and insulin and are developing complications.

Other Treatments

Your doctor will check your lipid profile and start you on medications to lower your LDL cholesterol below 100 mg/dl (optimally around 70 mg/dl) and triglycerides below 150 mg/dl. Your blood pressure should be consistently below 130/80, and if you are above this level, your doctor will start you on blood pressure medicines—usually an ACE inhibitor. You may also be prescribed a low-dose aspirin tablet daily.

Your doctor will also screen and treat for complications of diabetes as outlined in Chapters 3 and 4.

GLOSSARY

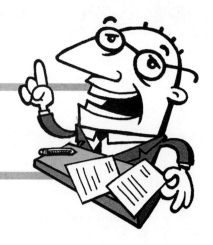

A1c *See* HbA1c.

acanthosis nigricans Dark velvety skin usually seen at the back of the neck or under armpit that is a sign of insulin resistance

Addison's disease Autoimmune damage to adrenal gland that results in deficiency of the stress hormone cortisol

alpha cells Cells in the islets of Langerhans in the pancreas that make glucagon

angina Pain in the chest, usually experienced during exercise, because of narrowing of the blood vessels that supply blood to the muscles of the heart

angiotensin converting enzyme (ACE) inhibitor a blood pressure medicine

angiotensin receptor blocker (ARB) a blood pressure medicine

antibodies Proteins made by the B cells of the immune system that stick to and remove bacteria and viruses

antioxidants Chemicals that neutralize the activity of reactive oxygen species inside cells

ARB Angiotensin receptor blocker; a blood pressure medicine

atherosclerosis Hardening and narrowing of blood vessels caused by fatty deposits

Atkins Diet A carbohydrate-restricted diet with most calories supplied by proteins and fats

autoantibodies Antibodies that the immune system mistakenly makes against its own body proteins

autoimmune injury An autoimmune disease that occurs when the body's immune system mistakenly attacks and destroys its own tissues. Examples include type 1 diabetes, celiac disease, and autoimmune thyroid diseases (Hashimoto's thyroiditis and Graves' disease).

autonomic neuropathy Injury of the autonomic nervous system (sympathetic and parasympathetic) that controls involuntary functions of the body such as blood pressure and gastrointestinal functions

autonomic symptoms Symptoms of shaking, sweating, and heart racing that occur with low glucose reactions

Bell's palsy A paralysis of the nerve supplying the muscles on one side of the face

beta cells Insulin-producing cells found in the islets of Langerhans within the pancreas

BMI Body mass index—a measure of obesity

calorie A unit of energy. In precise scientific terms, a kilocalorie (1,000 calories) is the energy required to raise the temperature of 1 liter of water by 1 degree centigrade.

carbohydrate (CHO) Food type—glucose, starches, and fiber are all carbohydrates

carbohydrate counting Estimating carbohydrate content of a food

carpal tunnel syndrome A condition that causes tingling, numbness, and weakness in the hand because of pinching of the median nerve at the wrist. One of the repetitive strain disorders that occurs more frequently in people with diabetes.

cataracts Clouding of the lens of the eye—occurs as part of the natural aging process but occurs earlier and more frequently in people with diabetes

CDE Certified Diabetes Educator

celiac disease An autoimmune disease of the small intestine that occurs in a susceptible individual in response to eating foods that contain gluten

Charcot's arthropathy Damage to a joint, usually the ankle or foot, in the presence of diabetic nerve damage (see Chapter 3)

cholesterol A steroid chemical used by the body to make hormones and a component of cell membranes

chylomicrons Particles that deliver fat and cholesterol from the small intestine to the liver

coronary artery disease Hardening of and narrowing of blood vessels of the heart by atheroma. The narrowing can limit blood flow, causing angina, or there can be a blockage causing a heart attack.

creatinine Chemical made by muscle and released into the blood. Creatinine is removed by the kidneys, and its level rises when there is kidney failure.

CSIRO (Commonwealth Scientific and Industrial Research Organization) Total Wellbeing Diet (Australian) Moderately high protein diet

dawn phenomenon Hormonal changes in the body that lead to increased insulin needs early in the morning (about 4 to 8 A.M.). In people with diabetes, glucose levels rise during this time if additional insulin is not provided.

diabetes mellitus or **diabetes** A disorder of elevated blood glucose because of absolute or relative deficiency of insulin

diabetes self-management education (DSME) The process of learning to take care of your diabetes

diabetic amyotrophy Diabetic nerve injury causing severe pain and weakness of the thigh

diabetic ketoacidosis (DKA) A condition where a lack of insulin leads to high levels of glucose, free fatty acids, and ketones. Untreated it can lead to coma.

dialysis An artificial kidney machine used when kidneys are no longer functioning

diuretic A medicine that makes you urinate more. Also called water pill. It is used to treat heart failure and high blood pressure.

Dupuytren's contractures Thickening and shrinking of the connective tissue of the hand so that the fingers get curved

endocrinologist A physician who specializes in the diseases of the hormone-producing glands of the body. Diabetes is a disease of the insulin-producing islets of Langerhans—an endocrine organ.

erectile dysfunction Inability to obtain and sustain an erection (impotence)

fiber A form of carbohydrate that is not digested by humans

frozen shoulder A condition where there is pain, stiffness, and loss of movement at the shoulder joint

fructosamine A measure of glucose coating of proteins in the blood, principally albumin. Fructosamine levels assess glucose control over the previous three weeks.

fructose A simple sugar that does not require insulin for its metabolism

gangrene Death of body tissue (for example, toes) due to lack of blood flow

gastroparesis Nerve damage to the stomach affecting its emptying

gestational diabetes Diabetes that first appears during pregnancy and most often disappears after delivery. Patients who get this are at increased risk of developing type 2 diabetes in the future.

glaucoma Increased fluid pressure inside the eye that if not treated leads to visual loss

glucagon A hormone produced by alpha cells in the islets that counteracts the effect of insulin and raises blood glucose. Glucagon injections are used in the treatment of severe hypoglycemia when the patient cannot take oral fast-acting carbohydrate.

glucose A simple sugar and an important energy source of the body

glycemic index The glucose rise of the food in question compared to the rise after eating a standard 50-gram glucose load

glycogen The main glucose storage form in the liver and muscles

glycohemoglobin *See* HbA1c.

Graves' disease An autoimmune disorder where an autoantibody causes the thyroid gland to make and release excessive amounts of thyroid hormone

Hashimoto's thyroiditis Immunological injury to the thyroid that frequently leads to low levels of thyroid hormone in the blood

HbA1c Also called A1c or glycohemoglobin. The amount of glucose attached to the hemoglobin inside the red cells (the "sugar attachment")—a measure of average glucose levels in the previous three months.

HDL Particles that carry cholesterol from the tissues to the liver. HDL cholesterol is referred to as the "good" cholesterol because generally higher levels are associated with a decreased risk of heart disease.

heart attack Acute blockage of a blood vessel that supplies blood to the heart muscles. It is a medical emergency because if the blockage is not cleared it will cause the area of the heart supplied by that blood vessel to die.

heart failure Inability of the heart to adequately pump blood to meet the body's needs. It occurs when there is damage to the heart valves or the heart muscles or both. Heart attack is a common cause of heart failure.

hemoglobin A1c *See* HbA1c.

high-density lipoproteins *See* HDL.

honeymoon phase The time after initial diagnosis of type 1 diabetes when the body still makes some insulin. The honeymoon phase ends when the patient is completely dependent on insulin given by injection.

hormone A chemical messenger released into the bloodstream

hyperosmolar coma Result of severely uncontrolled diabetes with glucose levels often over 800 mg/dl that untreated leads to severe dehydration and coma

hypertension High blood pressure

hypoglycemia Low blood glucose. Also called insulin reaction or insulin shock.

hypoglycemic unawareness Blunting of the ability to recognize low glucose reactions. This occurs in people who have diabetes for many years and in people who have very frequent low glucose reactions.

impaired fasting glucose (IFG) When the fasting glucose is not normal but is not in the diabetes range (100 to 125 mg/dl). Also called prediabetes.

impaired glucose tolerance (IGT) When the two-hour glucose level after drinking 75 grams of glucose is in the range of 140 to 199. Also called prediabetes.

impotence *See* erectile dysfunction.

incidence New cases of a disease in a population. *See also* prevalence.

insulin A hormone produced by the beta cells of the islets of Langerhans. It regulates the glucose levels in the blood. Insulin is needed to move glucose into muscles and fat cells and for storing glucose as glycogen in the liver and muscles.

insulin analogs Human insulin modified so as to alter its absorption after subcutaneous injection

insulin-dependent diabetes mellitus (IDDM) *See* type 1 diabetes.

insulin reaction *See* hypoglycemia.

insulin resistance Compared to insulin-sensitive people, insulin-resistant individuals need more insulin to have the same effect. Many people with type 2 diabetes

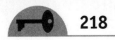

are insulin resistant. Obesity, especially around the waist, increases insulin resistance.

insulin resistant *See* insulin resistance.

insulin sensitive *See* insulin resistance.

intermittent claudication Pain in the calves or legs with walking, especially up hills, due to impaired blood flow to the legs and relieved by rest

islets of Langerhans Clusters of cells scattered throughout the pancreas that produce several hormones including insulin and glucagon

ketones Chemicals made when the body uses fat for energy. Can be used by tissues for energy. Excessive amounts are made when body is insulin deficient, leading to a condition called diabetic ketoacidosis or DKA.

kilocalorie Equal to 1,000 calories. *See also* calorie.

lactic acidosis A medical condition in which there is a buildup of lactic acid in the body. People who are at risk include those with liver, kidney, and heart failure.

lancet A fine, sharp-pointed needle for pricking the skin to get a blood sample for measuring glucose

LDL Particles that transport cholesterol to the peripheral tissues. They come in different sizes, and small LDL particles can infiltrate the blood vessel walls, damaging them and leading to atherosclerosis. LDL cholesterol is sometimes referred to as "bad" cholesterol.

lipid panel or profile Blood tests for levels of total cholesterol, triglycerides, HDL cholesterol, and LDL cholesterol

lipohypertrophy A buildup of fat under the skin leading to a lump, caused by repeated insulin injections at the same spot

lipoprotein particles Protein-coated particles of fat and cholesterol

low-density lipoproteins *See* LDL.

macroalbuminuria Albumin levels in the urine that signify worsening kidney damage (more than 300 mg/g creatinine)

macrosomia Abnormally large baby born to a diabetic mother. Poor glucose control is a risk factor for macrosomia.

macrovascular complications Diseases of the large blood vessels such as coronary artery disease

macular edema Swelling of the macula that occurs in people who have diabetic retinopathy. The macula is the region of the retina that is responsible for fine vision.

McDougall Diet Very low fat (less than 10 percent of daily calories) vegetarian diet

metabolism The process inside cells by which chemicals are changed to release their energy. For example, the metabolism of glucose to carbon dioxide and water releases energy for use by the cell.

microalbuminuria Albumin levels in the urine that signify early kidney damage (30 to 300 mg/g creatinine)

microvascular complications Diseases of the small blood vessels such as those in the retina, nerves, and kidney

monounsaturated fats Fats with one double carbon bond and found in olive oil, canola oil, and peanuts

myocardial infarction Medical term for heart attack. *See* heart attack.

necrobiosis lipoidica diabeticorum Skin condition seen on the front of the lower legs more commonly in patients with type 1 diabetes

nephropathy Disease of the kidney

neuroglycopenic symptoms Confusion, blurred vision, and irritability—symptoms that occur when the brain is starved of glucose

neuropathy Nerve damage

non-insulin-dependent diabetes mellitus *See* type 2 diabetes.

onychomycosis Fungal infection of the nails

ophthalmologist A physician who specializes in diseases of the eye

oral glucose tolerance test (OGTT) A test for diagnosing diabetes. The test is performed after an overnight fast. Seventy-five grams of glucose are consumed, and the blood glucose level is measured two hours later.

Ornish Diet Very low fat (less than 10 percent of daily calories) vegetarian diet allowing eggs and dairy products

palpitations Fast heart rate

pancreas A gland behind the lower part of the stomach that produces insulin, glucagon, and enzymes that aid digestion

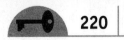

pancreatitis Inflammation of the pancreas

partially hydrogenated vegetable oils *See* trans fats.

plantar fasciitis Inflammation of the fascia of the foot

podiatrist A specialist in medical care and treatment of the foot

polycystic ovary syndrome (PCOS) A medical condition characterized by irregular menses and increased hairiness. Women with this condition have higher risk of diabetes.

polyunsaturated fats Fats with several double carbon bonds and found in vegetable oils such as safflower, corn, soybean, and sunflower and also in fish and seafood

postural hypotension Fall in blood pressure on sitting or standing resulting in symptoms of dizziness and light-headedness. Seen in patients with diabetic autonomic neuropathy.

prediabetes Glucose levels that are not normal but not high enough to be classified as diabetes. Individuals with glucoses in this range are at higher risk for heart disease and for future development of diabetes.

preeclampsia A serious condition of elevated blood pressure, urine protein loss, and kidney problems during pregnancy

prevalence Number of people affected by a disease in a population

priapism Prolonged erection—a side effect of medicines used for impotence

Pritikin Diet Very low fat (less than 10 percent of daily calories) nonvegetarian diet

proprioception Ability to sense the position of a joint or limb. In people with diabetes, nerve damage can affect proprioception, increasing risk of joint injury.

protein A component of food. Made up of chains of amino acids.

reactive oxygen species Chemicals containing oxygen that are made in response to metabolic reactions inside cells. Also called free radicals.

REE *See* resting energy expenditure.

resting energy expenditure (REE) energy expended at rest without exposure to cold

retina Light-sensitive layer at the back of the eye

retinal detachment Separation of part of the retina from the wall of the eye— results in vision loss

retinopathy Abnormalities of the blood vessels at the back of the eye due to diabetes. Background retinopathy is the early changes. Proliferative retinopathy is more severe changes that can lead to vision loss.

saturated fats Fats with no double carbon bonds and found in animal fats such as lard, butter, cheese, milk, meat, and coconut and palm kernel oil.

scleredema diabeticorum Itchy swelling and thickening of the skin of the shoulders and upper back that sometimes occurs in people with diabetes

shin spots Brown oval patches on the shins of people with diabetes

South Beach Diet High-protein diet with preferences for monounsaturated and polyunsaturated fats and limited low-glycemic carbohydrates

stroke Damage to the brain because of blockage or leaking of a blood vessel

subcutaneous injection Injection into the tissue beneath the skin

sugar alcohols Not as easily absorbed as regular sugar and so used as sweeteners in sugar-free food products such as chewing gum

symptoms The medical term for any sensation or feeling experienced by the patient because of an illness—for example, tingling in the feet might be a symptom of diabetic neuropathy

trans fats Partially hydrogenated plant oils that in the body raise LDL cholesterol and lower HDL cholesterol

transient ischemic attack (TIA) Neurological symptoms due to brief interruption of blood supply to a part of the brain, for example, weakness of an arm or leg or a problem speaking. Usually gets better in an hour but sometimes can last up to twenty-four hours. If the symptoms last more than twenty-four hours, it is referred to as a stroke.

trigger finger Momentary pain and catching of the finger or thumb as it is being straightened, caused by the narrowing of the snug tunnel that the tendons of the finger and thumb pass through

triglyceride A major energy source of the body stored in fat cells. It consists of glycerol attached to three fatty acid chains.

type 1 diabetes Previously called juvenile or insulin-dependent diabetes mellitus (IDDM). An autoimmune disorder with the immune system specifically destroying the beta cells of the islets of Langerhans.

type 2 diabetes Previously called non-insulin-dependent diabetes mellitus (NIDDM) or adult-onset diabetes. A disorder characterized by insulin resistance as well as impaired insulin secretion. Obesity is an important cause of acquired insulin resistance.

very low-density lipoproteins *See* VLDL.

VLDL Particles made in the liver containing mostly triglycerides and some cholesterol. They are responsible for transporting triglycerides to the fat cells.

Zone Diet Diet where every meal is 30 percent protein, 30 percent fat, and 40 percent carbohydrates

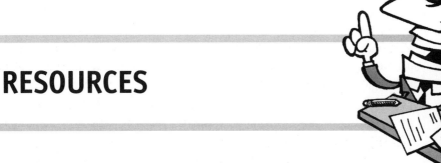

RESOURCES

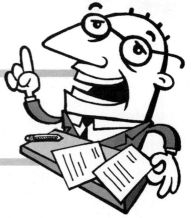

American Diabetes Association: diabetes.org

British Diabetes Association: diabetes.org.uk

Canadian Diabetes Association: diabetes.ca

Juvenile Diabetes Foundation: jdf.org

National Diabetes Information Clearinghouse (NDIC) at National Institutes of Health: http://diabetes.niddk.nih.gov/intro/index.htm

MedlinePlus website maintained by U.S. National Library of Medicine and National Institutes of Health (information on medical conditions, medical tests, and medications): nlm.nih.gov/medlineplus

- For information about different kinds of diabetes, check out the American Diabetes Association position paper on the diagnosis and classification of diabetes mellitus at http://care.diabetesjournals.org/cgi/reprint/26/suppl_1/s5.pdf (or key words on Google search: "diagnosis and classification of diabetes mellitus ADA").

- For a fact sheet about depression and diabetes from the National Institute of Mental Health, go to nimh.nih.gov/publicat/depdiabetes.cfm.

- Websites on diabetes complications: http://diabetes.niddk.nih.gov/complications/index.htm and http://diabetes.niddk.nih.gov/dm/pubs/complications_heart/index.htm.

- Information on dialysis can be found at the National Kidney Foundation website: kidney.org/atoz/atozItem.cfm?id=39.

- Information on nutritional supplements for use in diabetes is available at http://care.diabetesjournals.org/cgi/content/full/26/4/1277. Also look at the United States Pharmcopeia website at usp.org/aboutUSP.

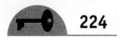

- Blood glucose awareness training—a program run by the University of Virginia to help people with type 1 diabetes to recognize, anticipate, and prevent extreme fluctuations in blood glucose levels: healthsystem.virginia .edu/bmc/bgathome/flash/index2.htm.

- Driving regulations for your state at the ADA website: diabetes.org/ advocacy-and-legalresources/discrimination/drivers/pvt-driverslicenses.jsp.

- The USDA National Nutrient Database for Standard Reference—Release 19 is a public reference database that gives comprehensive information about calories, carbohydrates, fats, proteins, potassium content, and sodium content for 7,293 foods and is free to download and use at ars.usda.gov. Also look at nal.usda.gov/fnic/databases.shtml.

- Websites where you can information on the glycemic index of foods: glycemicindex.com and mendosa.com/gilists.htm.

- The EPA website where you can get advice about mercury contamination of fish: http://epa.gov/waterscience/fish/advisory.html.

- The FDA has a website that explains how to use food label information: cfsan.fda.gov/~dms/foodlab.html.

- You can estimate your risk for heart disease using the ADA Diabetes Personal Health Decisions online questionnaire at diabetes.org/ diabetesPHD/default.jsp.

- The National Institutes of Health have information about healthy weight and how to achieve it at nhlbi.nih.gov/health/public/heart/obesity/lose_wt/ index.htm.

- To calculate your BMI and your energy needs, go to the Baylor College of Medicine website at bcm.edu/cnrc/caloriesneed.htm. You can also get a handout at the University of Arizona website at http://nutrition.arizona.edu/ new/files/01Calorie_Need_Estimates.pdf.

- For more information about the plate method of portion control, go to http://platemethod.com/publications.html.

- Comparison charts for the different insulin pumps can be found at diabetesnet.com/diabetes_technology/insulin_pump_models.php and integrateddiabetes.com/pump_c.shtml. The following website has links and lots of information about insulin pumps: insulin-pumpers.org/index.shtml.

- Go to the CDC website at cdc.gov/travel for the latest information on travel and to the TSA website at tsa.gov/travelers/airtravel/specialneeds/index .shtm for information regarding going through airport security.

- The International Diabetes Federation website at idf.org/home/index .cfm?node=10 has contact information for diabetes organizations in different countries.

- The CDC website has the recommendations for pneumonia and influenza immunization at cdc.gov/mmwR/preview/mmwrhtml/mm5343a2.htm.

- You can go to the American Medical Association website to get more information for advanced health directives: ama-assn.org/ama/pub/ category/14894.html#patients.

- The National Hospice and Palliative Care Organization (NHPCO) website has state-specific advance directives for download at nhpco.org/i4a/forms/ form.cfm?id=88.

- MedlinePlus has information and links to several other websites regarding diabetes and pregnancy at nlm.nih.gov/medlineplus/diabetesandpregnancy .html.

- The ADA has set out recommendations on how schools and day care centers should respond to children with diabetes and how to set up a Diabetes Health Care Plan for your child, available at http://care .diabetesjournals.org/cgi/reprint/25/suppl_1/s122.pdf.

- You can get trendy identification bracelets and necklaces that might appeal to children and adolescents at childrenwithdiabetes.com/d_06_700.htm.

- The Children with Diabetes and ADA websites have information about diabetes camping programs at childrenwithdiabetes.com/cgi-bin/cwdsearch .pl and diabetes.org/communityprograms-and-localevents/diabetescamps .jsp.

- Inject-Ease is a device for children who are frightened of needles: see the website palcolabs.com/section_products/injectease.html for details.

- Children with Diabetes offers an excellent website on all aspects of diabetes management in children at childrenwithdiabetes.com/index_cwd .htm.

- TrialNet is an NIH-funded organization that is coordinating research studies on the prevention of type 1 diabetes: diabetestrialnet.org.

- The National Diabetes Education Program has a series of booklets on how to assess your risk for type 2 diabetes and what you can do to prevent the disease, available for download or order at http://ndep.nih.gov/diabetes/ prev/prevention.htm.

REFERENCES

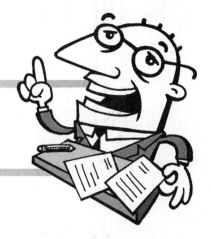

Chapter 1

American Diabetes Association. "Diagnosis and classification of diabetes mellitus." *Diabetes Care* 2007 Jan; 30 (Suppl 1): S42–47.

American Diabetes Association. "Screening for type 2 diabetes." *Diabetes Care* 2003 Jan; 26 (Suppl 1): S21–24.

Chapter 2

Atkinson MA, Eisenbarth GS. "Type 1 diabetes: new perspectives on disease pathogenesis and treatment." *Lancet* 2001 Jul 21; 358 (9277): 221–29. Review. Erratum in: *Lancet* 2001 Sep 1; 358 (9283): 766.

Atkinson MA, Maclaren NK. "The pathogenesis of insulin-dependent diabetes mellitus." *N Engl J Med* 1994 Nov 24; 331 (21): 1428–36.

Barroso I. "Genetics of type 2 diabetes." *Diabet Med* 2005 May; 22 (5): 517–35.

Herold KC, Hagopian W, Auger JA, Poumian-Ruiz E, Taylor L, Donaldson D, Gitelman SE, et al. "Anti-CD3 monoclonal antibody in new-onset type 1 diabetes mellitus." *N Engl J Med* 2002 May 30; 346 (22): 1692–98.

Scott LJ, Mohlke KL, Bonnycastle LL, Willer CJ, Li Y, Duren WL, Erdos MR, et al. "A genome-wide association study of type 2 diabetes in Finns detects multiple susceptibility variants." *Science* 2007 Jun 1; 316 (5829): 1341–45.

Voltarelli JC, Couri CE, Stracieri AB, Oliveira MC, Moraes DA, Pieroni F, Coutinho M, et al. "Autologous nonmyeloablative hematopoietic stem cell transplantation in newly diagnosed type 1 diabetes mellitus." *JAMA* 2007 Apr 11; 297 (14): 1568–76.

Chapter 3

Brownlee M. "The pathobiology of diabetic complications: a unifying mechanism." *Diabetes* 2005 Jun; 54 (6): 1615–25.

Buse JB, Ginsberg HN, Bakris GL, Clark NG, Costa F, Eckel R, Fonseca V, et al. "Primary prevention of cardiovascular diseases in people with diabetes mellitus: a scientific statement from the American Heart Association and the American Diabetes Association." *Diabetes Care* 2007 Jan; 30 (1): 162–72.

Caruso S, Rugolo S, Agnello C, Intelisano G, Di Mari L, Cianci A. "Sildenafil improves sexual functioning in premenopausal women with type 1 diabetes who are affected by sexual arousal disorder: a double-blind, crossover, placebo-controlled pilot study." *Fertil Steril* 2006 May; 85 (5): 1496–1501.

Ferris FL 3rd. "How effective are treatments for diabetic retinopathy?" *JAMA* 1993 Mar 10; 269 (10): 1290–91.

Hayden M, Pignone M, Phillips C, Mulrow C. "Aspirin for the primary prevention of cardiovascular events: a summary of the evidence for the U.S. Preventive Services Task Force." *Ann Intern Med* 2002 Jan 15; 136 (2): 161–72.

Rendell MS, Rajfer J, Wicker PA, Smith MD. "Sildenafil for treatment of erectile dysfunction in men with diabetes: a randomized controlled trial. Sildenafil Diabetes Study Group." *JAMA* 1999 Feb 3; 281 (5): 421–26.

Stuckey BG, Jadzinsky MN, Murphy LJ, Montorsi F, Kadioglu A, Fraige F, Manzano P, Deerochanawong C. "Sildenafil citrate for treatment of erectile dysfunction in men with type 1 diabetes: results of a randomized controlled trial." *Diabetes Care* 2003 Feb; 26 (2): 279–84.

Chapter 4

Anderson RJ, Freedland KE, Clouse RE, Lustman PJ. "The prevalence of comorbid depression in adults with diabetes: a meta-analysis." *Diabetes Care* 2001 Jun; 24 (6): 1069–78.

Rizza RA, Vigersky RA, Rodbard HW, Ladenson PW, Young WF Jr, Surks MI, Kahn R, Hogan PF. "A model to determine workforce needs for endocrinologists in the United States until 2020." *Diabetes Care* 2003 May; 26 (5): 1545–52.

Chapter 5

Rohlfing CL, Wiedmeyer HM, Little RR, England JD, Tennill A, Goldstein DE. "Defining the relationship between plasma glucose and HbA(1c): analysis of glucose profiles and HbA(1c) in the Diabetes Control and Complications Trial." *Diabetes Care* 2002 Feb; 25 (2): 275–78.

Chapter 6

Bode BW, Sabbah HT, Gross TM, Fredrickson LP, Davidson PC. "Diabetes management in the new millennium using insulin pump therapy." *Diabetes Metab Res Rev* 2002; 18 (Suppl 1): S14–20.

Khan A, Safdar M, Ali Khan MM, Khattak KN, Anderson RA. "Cinnamon improves glucose and lipids of people with type 2 diabetes." *Diabetes Care* 2003 Dec; 26 (12): 3215–18.

Kuchulakanti P, Waksman R. "Therapeutic potential of oral antiproliferative agents in the prevention of coronary restenosis." *Drugs* 2004; 64 (21): 2379–88.

Martin J, Wang ZQ, Zhang XH, Wachtel D, Volaufova J, Matthews DE, Cefalu WT. "Chromium picolinate supplementation attenuates body weight gain and increases insulin sensitivity in subjects with type 2 diabetes." *Diabetes Care* 2006 Aug; 29 (8): 1826–32.

Nissen SE, Wolski K. "Effect of rosiglitazone on the risk of myocardial infarction and death from cardiovascular causes." *N Engl J Med* 2007 May 21; [Epub ahead of print].

Sotaniemi EA, Haapakoski E, Rautio A. "Ginseng therapy in non-insulin-dependent diabetic patients." *Diabetes Care* 1995 Oct; 18 (10): 1373–75.

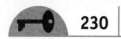
Takagi T, Yamamuro A, Tamita K, Yamabe K, Katayama M, Mizoguchi S, Ibuki M, et al. "Pioglitazone reduces neointimal tissue proliferation after coronary stent implantation in patients with type 2 diabetes mellitus: an intravascular ultrasound scanning study." *Am Heart J* 2003 Aug; 146 (2): E5.

UK Prospective Diabetes Study (UKPDS) Group. "Effect of intensive blood-glucose control with metformin on complications in overweight patients with type 2 diabetes (UKPDS 34)." *Lancet* 1998 Sep 12; 352 (9131): 854–65. Erratum in: *Lancet* 1998 Nov 7; 352 (9139): 1558.

UK Prospective Diabetes Study (UKPDS) Group. "Intensive bloodglucose control with sulphonylureas or insulin compared with conventional treatment and risk of complications in patients with type 2 diabetes (UKPDS 33)." *Lancet* 1998 Sep 12; 352 (9131): 837–53. Erratum in: *Lancet* 1999 Aug 14; 354 (9178): 602.

Vanschoonbeek K, Thomassen BJ, Senden JM, Wodzig WK, van Loon LJ. "Cinnamon supplementation does not improve glycemic control in postmenopausal type 2 diabetes patients." *J Nutr* 2006 Apr; 136 (4): 977–80.

Vuksan V, Sievenpiper JL, Xu Z, Wong EY, Jenkins AL, Beljan-Zdravkovic U, Leiter LA, Josse RG, Stavro MP. "Konjac-Mannan and American ginseng: emerging alternative therapies for type 2 diabetes mellitus." *J Am Coll Nutr* 2001 Oct; 20 (5 Suppl): 370S–80S; discussion 381S–83S.

Chapter 7

Austin EJ, Deary IJ. "Effects of repeated hypoglycemia on cognitive function: a psychometrically validated reanalysis of the Diabetes Control and Complications Trial data." *Diabetes Care* 1999 Aug; 22 (8): 1273–77.

Briscoe VJ, Davis SN. "Hypoglycemia in type 1 and type 2 diabetes." *Physiology, Pathophysiology, and Management Clinical Diabetes* 2006; 24: 115–21.

de Galan BE, Schouwenberg BJ, Tack CJ, Smits P. "Pathophysiology and management of recurrent hypoglycaemia and hypoglycaemia unawareness in diabetes." *Neth J Med* 2006; 64: 269–79.

Jacobson AM, et al. "Effects of intensive and conventional treatment on cognitive function twelve years after the completion of the Diabetes Control and Complications Trial (DCCT)." Abstract Number 750232, presented at the American Diabetes Association's 66th Annual Scientific Sessions held in Washington, D.C., June 13, 2006.

Chapter 8

American Diabetes Association. "Nutrition recommendations and interventions for diabetes." *Diabetes Care* 2007 Jan; 30 (Suppl 1): S48–S65.

American Diabetes Association Task Force for Writing Nutrition Principles and Recommendations for the Management of Diabetes and Related Complications. "American Diabetes Association position statement: evidence-based nutrition principles and recommendations for the treatment and prevention of diabetes and related complications." *J Am Diet Assoc* 2002 Jan; 102 (1): 109–18.

de Lorgeril M, Salen P, Martin JL, Monjaud I, Delaye J, Mamelle N. "Mediterranean diet, traditional risk factors, and the rate of cardiovascular complications after myocardial infarction: final report of the Lyon Diet Heart Study." *Circulation* 1999 Feb 16; 99 (6): 779–85.

Foster-Powell K, Holt SHA, and Brand-Miller JC. "International table of glycemic index and glycemic load values." *American Journal of Clinical Nutrition* 2002; 76 (1): 5–56.

Turpeinen O, Karvonen MJ, Pekkarinen M, Miettinen M, Elosuo R, Paavilainen E. "Dietary prevention of coronary heart disease: the Finnish Mental Hospital Study." *Int J Epidemiol* 1979 Jun; 8 (2): 99–118.

Chapter 9

American College of Sports Medicine and American Diabetes Association joint position statement. "Diabetes mellitus and exercise." *Med Sci Sports Exerc* 1997; 29: i–vi.

Perkins BA, Riddell MC. "Type 1 diabetes and exercise: using the insulin pump to maximum advantage." *Canadian Journal of Diabetes* 2006; 30; 72–79.

Sigal RJ, Castaneda-Sceppa C, Kenny GP, White RD, Wasserman DH. "Physical/exercise and type 2 diabetes." *Diabetes Care* 2006; 29: 1433–38.

Walsh J, Roberts R. *Pumping Insulin*. 3rd ed. San Diego, CA: Torrey Pines Press; 2000.

Wasserman DH, Zinman B. "Exercise in individuals with IDDM." *Diabetes Care* 1994; 17: 924–37.

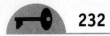

Chapter 10

Bravata DM, Sanders L, Huang J, Krumholz HM, Olkin I, Gardner CD, Bravata DM. "Efficacy and safety of low-carbohydrate diets." *JAMA* 2003 Apr 9; 289 (14): 1837–50.

Buchwald H, Avidor Y, Braunwald E, Jensen MD, Pories W, Fahrbach K, Schoelles K. "Bariatric surgery: a systematic review and meta-analysis." *JAMA* 2004; 292: 1724–37. Review. Erratum in: *JAMA* 2005; 293: 1728.

Colquitt J, Clegg A, Loveman E, Royle P, Sidhu MK. "Surgery formorbid obesity." *Cochrane Database Syst Rev* 2005 Oct 19; 4: CD003641.

DPP Research Group. "Description of lifestyle intervention." *Diabetes Care* 2002; 25: 2165–71.

Haddock CK, Poston WS, Dill PL, Foreyt JP, Ericsson M. "Pharmacotherapy for obesity: a quantitative analysis of four decades of published randomized clinical trials." *Int J Obes Relat Metab Disord* 2002 Feb; 26 (2): 262–73.

Heymsfield SB, van Mierlo CA, van der Knaap HC, Heo M, Frier HI. "Weight management using a meal replacement strategy: meta and pooling analysis from six studies." *Int J Obes Relat Metab Disord* 2003 May; 27 (5): 537–49.

James WP, Astrup A, Finer N, Hilsted J, Kopelman P, Rossner S, Saris WH, Van Gaal LF. "Effect of sibutramine on weight maintenance after weight loss: a randomised trial. STORM Study Group. Sibutramine Trial of Obesity Reduction and Maintenance." *Lancet* 2000 Dec 23–30; 356 (9248): 2119–25.

Lean M, Lara J. "ABC of obesity: Strategies for preventing obesity." *BMJ* 2006; 333 (7575): 959–62.

Li Z, Maglione M, Tu W, Mojica W, Arterburn D, Shugarman LR, Hilton L, et al. "Meta analysis: pharmacologic treatment of obesity." *Ann Intern Med* 2005 Apr 5; 142 (7): 532–46.

Low AK, Bouldin MJ, Sumrall CD, Loustalot FV, Land KK. "A clinician's approach to medical management of obesity." *Am J Med Sci* 2006 Apr; 331 (4): 175–82.

Maggard MA, Shugarman LR, Suttorp M, Maglione M, Sugerman HJ, Livingston EH, Nguyen NT, et al. "Meta-analysis: surgical treatment of obesity." *Ann Intern Med* 2005 Apr 5; 142 (7): 547–59.

Miffin MD, St Jeor ST, Hill LA, Scott BJ, Daugherty SA, Koh YO. "A new predictive equation for resting energy expenditure in healthy individuals." *Am J Clin Nutr* 1990; 51: 241–47.

Nordmann AJ, Nordmann A, Briel M, Keller U, Yancy WS, Brehm BJ, Bucher HC. "Effects of low-carbohydrate vs low-fat diets on weight loss and cardiovascular risk factors: a meta-analysis of randomized controlled trials." *Arch Intern Med* 2006; 166: 285–93.

Padwal R, Li SK, Lau DC. "Long-term pharmacotherapy for obesity and overweight." *Cochrane Database Syst Rev* 2004; 3: CD004094.

Rothacker DQ. "Five-year self-management of weight using meal replacements: comparison with matched controls in rural Wisconsin." *Nutrition* 2000; 16 (5): 344–48.

Sjostrom L, Lindroos AK, Peltonen M, Torgerson J, Bouchard C, Carlsson B, Dahlgren S, et al. "Lifestyle, diabetes, and cardiovascular risk factors 10 years after bariatric surgery." *N Engl J Med* 2004 Dec 23; 351 (26): 2683–93.

Chapter 11

Burnett JC. "Long- and short-haul travel by air: issues for people with diabetes on insulin." *J Travel Med* 2006 Sep–Oct; 13 (5): 255–60.

Chapter 13

American Diabetes Association. "Position statement. Gestational diabetes mellitus." *Diabetes Care* 2003; 26 (Suppl 1): S103–5.

American Diabetes Association. "Preconception care of women with diabetes." *Diabetes Care* 2004; 27 (Suppl 1): S76–78.

Coustan DR, Carpenter MW. "The diagnosis of gestational diabetes." *Diabetes Care* 1998; 21 (Suppl 2): B5–8.

Gabbe SG, Graves CR. "Management of diabetes mellitus complicating pregnancy." *Obstet Gynecol* 2003; 102: 857–68.

Jovanovic L, Nakai Y. "Successful pregnancy in women with type 1 diabetes: from preconception through postpartum care." *Endocrinol Metab Clin North Am* 2006; 35: 79–97.

Price N, Bartlett C, Gillmer M. "Use of insulin glargine during pregnancy: a case-control pilot study." *BJOG* 2007 Apr; 114 (4): 453–57.

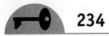

Xiang AH, Peters RK, Kjos SL, Marroquin A, Goico J, Ochoa C, Kawakubo M, Buchanan TA. "Effect of pioglitazone on pancreatic beta-cell function and diabetes risk in Hispanic women with prior gestational diabetes." *Diabetes* 2006 Feb; 55 (2): 517–22.

Zarzycki W, Zieniewicz M. "Reproductive disturbances in type 1 diabetic women." *Neuro Endocrinol Lett* 2005 Dec; 26 (6): 733–38.

Chapter 14

American Association of Diabetes Educators. "Management of children with diabetes in the school setting." *Diabetes Educ* 2000; 26: 32–35.

American Diabetes Association. "Diabetes care at diabetes camps." *Diabetes Care* 2007 Jan; 30 (Suppl 1): S74–76.

American Diabetes Association. "Diabetes care in the school and day care setting." *Diabetes Care* 2007 Jan; 30 (Suppl 1): S66–73.

Bloomgarden ZT. "Type 2 diabetes in the young: the evolving epidemic." *Diabetes Care* 2004 Apr; 27 (4): 998–1010.

Silverstein J, Klingensmith G, Copeland K, Plotnick L, Kaufman F, Laffel L, Deeb L, et al. "Care of children and adolescents with type 1 diabetes: a statement of the American Diabetes Association." *Diabetes Care* 2005 Jan; 28 (1): 186–212.

Chapter 15

Benbow SJ, Walsh A, Gill GV. "Diabetes in institutionalised elderly people: a forgotten population?" *BMJ* 1997 Jun 28; 314 (7098): 1868–69.

Gregg EW, Engelgau MM, Narayan V. "Complications of diabetes in elderly people." *BMJ* 2002 Oct 26; 325 (7370): 916–17.

Chapter 16

Nathan DM, Buse JB, Davidson MB, Heine RJ, Holman RR, Sherwin R, Zinman B. "Management of hyperglycemia in type 2 diabetes: a consensus algorithm for the initiation and adjustment of therapy: a consensus statement from the American Diabetes Association and the European Association for the Study of Diabetes." *Diabetes Care* 2006; 29: 1963–72.

Sherwin RS, Anderson RM, Buse JB, Chin MH, Eddy D, Fradkin J, Ganiats TG, et al. "The prevention or delay of type 2 diabetes." *Diabetes Care* 2003; 26 (Suppl 1): S62–69.

INDEX

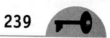

ABOUT THE AUTHOR

Dr. Umesh Masharani is a clinical professor of medicine in the division of endocrinology and metabolism and associate chief in the diabetes clinic at the University of California at San Francisco (UCSF). In addition to seeing patients and teaching, he does clinical research in diabetes. Dr. Masharani got his medical degree at the Middlesex Hospital, London, and completed his fellowship in endocrinology at UCSF.